Hippocrates

Medical Insights to Promote Wellbeing

This series collects books on health and wellbeing topics addressed to lay persons, patients, families, and patients associations. Healthcare providers also benefit from this series, in particular GPs interested in improving their doctor-patient communication.

Designed to be accessible and informative, it helps readers to understand complex medical and health topics thus promoting healthy habits and well-being for all at all ages.

The Hippocrates series will include volumes on:

- Women's health
- Men's health
- Sexual and reproductive Health
- Maternal and newborn Health
- Child and adolescent Health
- Addiction (drugs, alcohol, tobacco, …)
- Aging
- Cardiovascular diseases
- Dermatology
- Diabetes
- Disability
- Environment and Health
- Mental Health
- Nutrition – Eating disorders
- Obesity
- Oncology
- Prevention
- Rehabilitation
- Viruses – Immunization – Vaccines – Infectious Diseases
- Wellbeing

Authored by medical experts from around the world, the Hippocrates books Series break down barriers and make medical and health knowledge more accessible.

Val Wilson

Diabetes Ancient and Modern

The Evolution of Diabetes as a Metabolic Disease

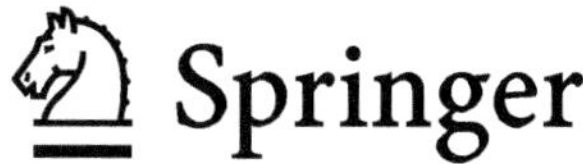

Val Wilson
Independent Diabetes Writer/Researcher
Kent, UK

ISSN 3091-2679 ISSN 3091-2687 (electronic)
Hippocrates
ISBN 978-3-032-12453-1 ISBN 978-3-032-12454-8 (eBook)
https://doi.org/10.1007/978-3-032-12454-8

This Springer imprint is published by the registered company Springer Nature Switzerland AG
The registered company address is: Gewerbestrasse 11, 6330 Cham, Switzerland

For Neil, without whom this book would not have been possible.

Introduction

Over the past two centuries, we have learned that diabetes is a complex disease with several root causes. It finds its place in an ancient Egyptian papyrus of 1500 B.C. as a disease characterised by 'too great emptying of urine'. Observing that it attracted ants, Indian physicians named it *Madhumeha*—honey-like urine, with the great Indian doctor Sushruta and the surgeon Charaka recognising that there were two different kinds of diabetes in 400–500 A.D.

Diabetes has been recognised for three millennia, with physician Aretaeus of Cappadocia (a historical region of central Turkey) giving recorded descriptions of the condition in the first century A.D. The great Persian physician Avicenna (980–1037 A.D.) offered his patients herbal concoctions as a remedy for the excretion of sweet urine. It was not until the eighteenth century that the condition became known as diabetes *mellitus*—the Latin tern for sweet like honey.

The tenacious search for an effective treatment finally arrived with the miracle discovery of insulin in the early twentieth century. Despite this, it was later realised that although patients were living longer with a way to lower sugar (glucose) levels, this did not mean these levels were normal. Over time, many people taking insulin developed serious secondary health conditions.

We now know that diabetes mellitus occurs when the body cannot use glucose for energy due to a lack of insulin. Insulin is a hormone produced by specialised cells in the pancreas, an organ in the abdomen. The role of insulin is to allow glucose (a type of sugar) in the blood to enter cells, providing them with the fuel to function. When insulin cannot work properly, glucose accumulates in the blood, eventually causing serious health problems. A lack of effective insulin is responsible for the development of diabetes mellitus.

There are three main types of diabetes mellitus: type 1 diabetes, type 2 diabetes and gestational diabetes, occurring in pregnancy. There is also a state before the diagnosis of type 2 diabetes, known as prediabetes:

- Type 1 diabetes is a disease where the body's immune system repeatedly attacks and destroys insulin-producing cells in the pancreas.
- Prediabetes describes blood glucose levels that are higher than normal, but not high enough to be diagnosed as type 2 diabetes.
- Type 2 diabetes is also known as insulin resistance, meaning that the body can no longer use or produce insulin effectively.

Characterised by prolonged high blood glucose levels, prediabetes is a condition that occurs before type 2 diabetes is diagnosed, so it will be included as type 2 diabetes, unless otherwise stated. Both types of diabetes have the same symptoms, but each has its own causes and treatments.

Type 1 diabetes, formerly known as insulin-dependent childhood onset diabetes results from major destruction of the insulin-producing cells of the pancreas. Some cells remain, but not enough insulin can be produced to maintain normal blood glucose levels. The exact reason the immune system attacks these cells is still being investigated, but a combination of genetic and environmental factors, such as viral infections, alter the composition of gut bacteria, and specific dietary components, each contributing to type 1 diabetes onset.

Type 2 diabetes was formerly known as non-insulin-dependent, or adult-onset diabetes. When glucose-lowering medication becomes less effective after a number of years, insulin is required to manage blood glucose levels. Type 2 diabetes occurs in 95% of cases, usually diagnosed in people who are over 45 years of age, but this condition is now also increasingly seen in children and young people as a result of an inactive lifestyle with little or no exercise, and/or a diet high in starches and sugars.

FACT
Current estimates of UK sugar intake show that school-age children and teenagers are consuming three times more sugar each day than is recommended. Adults are consuming twice the maximum recommended intake of sugar per day (National Diet and Nutritional Survey Programme).

We are currently in the midst of a diabetes epidemic, although almost half of all global type 2 diabetes cases remain undiagnosed because there are no specific symptoms. This means that any secondary health problems—chronic complications, such as eye, kidney, and heart disease—resulting from prolonged high glucose levels will also not be detected. Globally, an estimated 415 million people have type 2 diabetes (International Diabetes Federation, 2021). This is expected to rise to 642 million by 2040.

In the twenty-first century, those developing diabetes are the most fortunate in history. A diagnosis of diabetes brings with it a complete change in lifestyle—whether this is the steep learning curve of type 1 diabetes requiring daily insulin replacement, or type 2, with necessary close attention to a diet, exercise and glucose-lowering medicine regimen. If managed well, the individual can lead a normal, long and fulfilling life with the understanding and treatment advances we now have at our fingertips. However, there is global disparity, and not everyone has access to this level of diabetes care.

The advances in diabetes care and self-management technology are the result of a long tenacious history of guesswork, assumption and perseverance. We are still searching for a cure.

About This Book

Diabetes Ancient and Modern: The Evolution of Diabetes as a Metabolic Disease explores a comprehensive history of this condition. We begin with the first recognition of frequent urination and a raging thirst in ancient Egypt that characterises high glucose levels. Ancient medical knowledge also emerged in China, India, Persia, Greece and Rome, describing the appearance of two types of disease with similar symptoms—one a wasting disease and death sentence affecting the young, the other affecting older, sedentary individuals and the richer classes.

Without an effective treatment or cure, those developing diabetes relied on herbal and plant remedies to ease their symptoms. The impasse in medical advancement during the Middle Ages meant that little was achieved to find the cause of diabetes, or any effective treatment. Despite this, modest advances in knowledge and understanding were achieved in the East, Persia, Byzantine and parts of Europe, where diabetes was believed to be a disease of the kidneys and bladder, due to the vast quantities of urine passed by patients.

Some scientific advances in the testing of blood and urine allowed diabetes to be confirmed, and managed with starvation and undernutrition treatments, which had some effect, but were unsustainable. A renewed interest in what caused diabetes emerged with the widespread accessibility of the printed word from 1440. Galen's theory of imbalance in the body as the reason for disease was challenged, and the cause of diabetes continued to be investigated as scientific method overtook subjective observations.

The scientific age pushed chemical analysis to detect health and disease to the forefront, identifying glucose as the sugar present in the blood and urine of people with diabetes. Experimentation now pointed to the pancreas as the organ responsible for the disease. These revelations became the new science of endocrinology (the pancreas being an endocrine gland), with further advancement revealing that diabetes is due to a lack of the hormone, insulin.

The breakthrough discovery of insulin in 1921 revolutionised the treatment of type 1 diabetes. However, living longer allowed complications associated with high glucose levels to develop. This book considers the historical understanding of diabetes complications as doctors tried their utmost to treat patients with these problems. There was no commonplace urine or blood self-monitoring, or appropriate adjustment of insulin dosages, so diabetes management for the medic was a rather hit and miss affair.

Type 2 diabetes remained in the shadows as far as treatment advances were concerned, until the advent of metformin; although this was first mentioned in scientific literature as a blood-glucose lowering agent in 1922, it did not become widely available as a treatment until the 1950s. Further advances in the understanding and treatment of diabetes led to the development of blood glucose monitoring meters, home urine tests, specially tailored carbohydrate diets and the understanding that controlling glucose is the key to a healthy life with diabetes.

There followed the introduction of insulin pump therapy in the late 1970s for the continuous delivery of insulin under the skin in type 1 diabetes, designed to mimic an artificial pancreas. Pancreatic transplantation research advanced to stop the insulin-producing cells of the pancreas from being destroyed.

A continuous glucose self-monitoring device became available in the 1990s, and now, both type 1 and type 2 diabetes patients can wear a small glucose sensor to monitor their diabetes. The recent introduction of weight loss injections to effectively treat obesity-related type 2 diabetes allows many people to now live diabetes-free, although these treatments are not available to all: global disparities in diabetes care is examined in the final chapter.

Contents

About the Author

Val Wilson is a Fellow of the Royal Society of Public Health. She has been an academic for over 30 years, with a doctorate in Diabetes Health Education, and a master's in Diabetes Health Education and Health Promotion. As a specialist in this field, she has advised the Government and the health service on diabetes strategies, and conducted many studies looking at how and why people self-manage their diabetes. She has also carried out more than 10 years of voluntary work with a diabetes charity, and published widely on all aspects of living with, and caring for people with diabetes.

Her interest in the history of diabetes comes from having had very unpredictable type 1 diabetes for almost 50 years; this is difficult to control and manage.

Her mission is to inform, educate and support others with diabetes, their physicians and carers, to achieve a good quality of life with the condition.

International Diabetes Federation (2021) 'Diabetes now affects 1 in 10 adults worldwide'. https://idf.org/news/diabetes-now-affects-one-in-10-adults-worldwide/

1

Two Diseases with Similar Symptoms

Mankind turned from a roaming hunter-gatherer society to permanent settlements with the development of farming. Farming enabled larger concentrations of people to be established in villages that ultimately grew into towns and cities. Food was easier to gather via farming, affording more free time for individuals to become specialists in crafts, such as pottery, metal smelting, weaving and arts. As farming developed, so too did the specialisation of crops; this included growing specific medical herbs and plants to use in remedies to treat ill health. Individuals with herbal knowledge handed remedies down by word of mouth, and later by the written word. This was the foundation of what we call medicine today.

Medical knowledge tended to remain with one family in a village, and these skills and this experience were not shared with others until they could be recorded. This meant that different cultures were unable to adopt these practices into their own way of thinking, resulting in a gradual spread of medical knowledge. As medical practices were documented, libraries became established so the knowledge could be shared and then built upon by any culture. Diabetes as a medical condition was not known in ancient times, although descriptions of symptoms found in early accounts can be recognised as diabetes.

V. Wilson, *Diabetes Ancient and Modern*, Hippocrates,
https://doi.org/10.1007/978-3-032-12454-8_1

Ancient China

Ancient Chinese culture followed Taoist principles to prevent illness; physicians commonly used drugs such as opium, acupuncture remedies and massage to treat disease. It is also documented in 500 B.C. that finely powdered jade was swallowed to slow the ageing process and protect the body against the diminishing effects of diseases such as diabetes; with belief in an old Chinese saying (Holmes 1997):

> He who swallows jade will live as long as jade.

Chinese physician *Huang-Di* described diabetes in the *Huang Di Nei Jing* (*The Yellow Emperor's Classic of Internal Medicine*) written during the Hang Dynasty in 200 B.C. (Maoshing 1995). Part of this book, *Suwen* (*The Book of Plain Questions*), defines extreme emaciation in end-stage type 1 diabetes, as 'xiago ke' and 'fei xiao', which translate as 'wasting and thirsting', and 'xiao zhong' meaning 'excessive eating' (Dharmananda 2002). This appears to describe excessive hunger associated with untreated type 1 diabetes, where body cells are starved of glucose for fuel in the absence of enough insulin.

The *Suwen* (200 B.C.) also describes a disease characterised by the excretion of large quantities of urine containing sugar (Maoshing 1995). The symptoms of the condition are cited as rapid weight loss, which strongly suggests type 1 diabetes. Consistent with Greek and Indian thinking, physicians in ancient China also thought type 2 diabetes was caused by a rich, unhealthy diet as this condition mainly affected the well-off (Hong-Yen and Peacher 1978). *The Book of Plain Questions* suggests that diabetes results:

> When a person has eaten too much greasy and sweet food, the body produces dry-heat evils which causes qi to stay in the middle burner of the body until finally the qi flows upward and spills over resulting in diabetes.

Symptoms

Oriental medicines based in China spread to all areas of the Orient via trade routes. Like the ancient Indians, Chinese and Japanese physicians also documented the sweetness of diabetic urine which is said to have 'attracted dogs' (Hong-Yen and Peacher 1978). Medical practitioners found that the blood of patients with diabetes contained a level of sweetness, seeing that people with the condition had boils as a consequence, and warning signs similar to *renal* (kidney) *tuberculosis*. This now rare disease echoes the onset of type 1 diabetes: both conditions predominantly affect young adults, cause general ill health, weight loss, and frequent urination and pain in the bladder (Schaaf 2009). As with the rare condition, *diabetes insipidus*, in cases of renal tuberculosis there is no sweetness in the urine.

Chinese physicians noted excessive weight loss, thirst, hunger and frequent urination in cases of type 1 diabetes, and classified these symptoms under one of four disharmony patterns of the temperament (Hong-Yen and Peacher 1978). This reflected the common understanding at that time of an imbalance within the four humours of the body. An imbalance in body fluids was generally felt to be the cause of diabetes, associated with poor diet and an unhealthy environment (Zhu et al. 1983).

Yin and yang represent opposing factors in Chinese medicine: the yin-yang principle states that everything that exists is composed of opposite but equally reliant elements, for example, yin and yang, day and night.

Chinese physicians did not share the commonly held belief that diabetes was a disease of the kidneys. Negative external factors were believed to impair the function of the body's organs: type 1 diabetes resulted when the metabolic rate in the stomach changed, increasing the appetite. The kidneys then failed to separate the body fluids from the urine to be expelled, resulting in frequent passing of sweet urine. As the disease progressed, the deficiency of yin also damaged the qi (life force) and the yang, upsetting the relationship between yin and yang in the body (Zhu et al. 1983).

Treatments

Traditional Chinese medicine based and still bases treatments on easing the patient's symptoms, patterns of imbalance and areas of deficiency. In around 200 A.D. the *Jing Gui Yao Lue* medical text documents two traditional formulas still used today in China and Japan to treat diabetes (Hong-Yen and Peacher 1978). Ba Wei Di Huang Tang is recommended for frailty, tiredness and the production of large quantities of urine soon after water is drunk. Bai Hu Jia Ren Shen Tang is popular in Japan today, especially for the treatment of obesity and type 2 diabetes; this formula was used in ancient China to treat newly diagnosed diabetes (Dharmananda 2002).

Management of Diabetes

To manage diabetes effectively, Chinese physicians emphasised the need for a good diet. This referred to the amount of energy certain foods could provide—energy meaning how they made you feel, rather than their dietary value. People with diabetes were advised to add certain foods to their diet, such as spinach for its cooling, strengthening and thirst-quenching abilities, and celery as a boost for the kidneys, along with winter melon, which was believed to reduce the sweetness of the blood and urine (Mukherjee et al. 2006).

In China and Japan, ginseng (man-shaped root) was and still is a commonly used medicinal herb, believed to 'improve diabetes' by 'stimulating the debilitated' (Hikino 1991). Taken on its own or in a combination of other herbs, ginseng is used to restore the yang quality and was used to treat the symptoms of diabetes, including boils, frailty, tiredness, high levels of sweetness, sickness, frequent urination and sores (Ng and Yeung 1982).

Other herbs often used to treat and manage glucose levels in diabetes included bitter melon, onion, garlic and fenugreek to bring glucose levels down after meals, and the bark of the ginkgo biloba tree, to improve blood flow to the extremities (Hikino 1991). Although still beneficial to people with diabetes today, these herbs do not have a marked effect on high glucose levels.

Atherosclerosis describes fatty deposits on the artery walls. Ginseng was felt to improve this condition and several long-term complications of diabetes, namely heart disease, impotence (erectile dysfunction), intestinal complaints, diabetic diarrhoea and constipation (Ng and Yeung 1982). Modern research shows that ginseng does indeed possess these healing effects.

Extracts of high-quality ginseng (Panax ginseng) improve endocrine system function—a network of glands that produce and release hormones to regulate bodily functions, and blood glucose control in people with diabetes (Ng and Yeung 1982).

Ancient India

Indian medicine was influenced by the Persians, Greeks and Chinese (Nutton 2005). The *Ayurveda*—Sanskrit for 'life knowledge'—is the oldest body of literature in Hinduism (900 B.C.) which underpins the tradition of Ayurvedic medicine, placing great emphasis on balancing the mind, body and spirit to create inner harmony and equilibrium (Kutumbian 2005; Gearson 1993).

Sickness, disease and ill health were believed to be due to a disruption in one of the five elements making up the body: space, air, water, fire and earth.

Righting the imbalance relied on diet, natural cures and herbs tailored to the individual's body shape to restore stability, and the disease would pass (Kutumbian 2005). This belief is similar to that of the Greeks, who also believed the cause of illness was associated with fire, air, earth and water.

Symptoms

Ancient Indian texts described diabetes in some detail in 300 B.C., naming it 'Madhumeha' (honey-like urine), the urine being sticky to the touch and tasting sweet (Kutumbian 2005; Frank 1957). This shows recognition of the presence of sugar (glucose) in the urine. Indian physicians treated high glucose levels with plant medicines, diet and rigorous exercise. Two particular plants have been used for centuries in India to treat excess sweetness within the body: Gymnema sylvestre is a plant native to the tropical forests of India; and Pterocarpus is extracted from the Pterocarpus marsupium plant (Murray 1995).

Indians noted the passing of large amounts of dilute urine by those afflicted with diabetes. Physicians also documented that their patients complained of experiencing a sweet taste in the mouth; an unquenchable thirst (known medically as *polydipsia*); a loss of appetite; regular vomiting; drying [dehydration] and boils (Kutumbian 2005).

Diabetes was described by three distinguished Indian physicians, Charaka, Sushruta and Vaghbata, who documented the sweet taste of the patient's urine and observed that ants and flies were drawn to the sugary fluid (Dwivedi and Dwivedi 2007). There are no firm dates when these physicians were practising, although documentary evidence reports Sushruta as a renowned surgeon teaching and practising medicine in Kashi around 600 B.C., some 700 years previous to other reports.

Charaka was an Indian physician who encouraged the use of an asphalt mineral pitch obtained from very old rotted plant matter—known as Shilajit—to cure most diseases, including the prevention and treatment of diabetes (Dwivedi and Dwivedi 2007).

The Indian book of medicine *Materia Medica* (volume II) states that mineral-rich Shilajit can be effective in cases of diabetes for renewing spiritual and sexual energy (Nadkarmi 2005). Shilajit was also documented in the *Materia Medica* as relieving the symptoms of health issues associated with diabetes, such as impotence, chronic fatigue and nerve diseases, although there is no indication that concentrated minerals derived from old plant matter have any marked effect on blood glucose.

Sushruta recognised that diabetes mainly affected older, overweight individuals with an inactive lifestyle. He also saw that a different kind of diabetes affected people who were not overweight, bringing an early death—thought to be the first recognition between type 1 and type 2 diabetes. In his book *Ayur-Veda*, Sushruta showed his astute awareness of symptoms, writing of type 1 diabetes (Gearson 1993):

> When the doctor states that a man suffers from honey urine, he has also declared him incurable… sweet is the urine, the sweat and the phlegm.

Sushruta clearly links these symptoms with type 1 diabetes, although this is also the case with uncontrolled type 2 diabetes. With no available cure, patients with type 2 diabetes eventually died of high blood glucose levels—known medically as *hyperglycaemia*, and associated complications, such as heart disease.

Tasting a patient's urine as a means of diagnosis was commonplace. It is also the case that if glucose concentration is high enough in the blood that it spills over into the urine for excretion, glucose is also high in every body fluid, such as saliva in the mouth. The above quoted passage from the *Ayur-Veda* shows that for patients with untreated diabetes, physicians were aware that body fluids contained a level of sweetness, and that Sushruta was one of these trying to right this imbalance.

Treatments

Rather than the common theory that kidney disease was to blame, Sushruta believed diabetes was a disorder of the blood, brought about due to imbalance within the body and taking in large amounts of fluid. He prescribed astringents (Gearson 1993)—substances that cause body tissues to contract or shrink. Similar to modern ways of thinking, Sushruta advised his patients how to manage an excess of sweetness with diet and exercise. His opinion of type 2 diabetes being very common in ancient India is now true of this condition globally, making up 95% of cases.

Complications

Without an effective treatment, many people with diabetes didn't live long enough for the complications of long-term high blood glucose to develop. A lack of understanding that too much glucose is key to the development of chronic diabetes complications, such as eye, kidney, nerve and heart disease, was seldom documented in ancient records. As such, secondary conditions attributed to having diabetes are rarely mentioned (Bridgewater 2001).

With this in mind, it is extraordinary that Sushruta was recognised for his method of treating cataracts, an extremely common eye condition today in people with diabetes (Kansupada and Sassani 1997).

Today we recognise that diabetes and high blood glucose levels have a detrimental effect on all body structures, such as blood vessels, nerves, muscles, tendons, organs and bones. In fact, anywhere that blood flows in the body can be permanently altered at a cellular level by high blood glucose. It is usual that micro-changes in the small blood vessels of the eyes, nerves and kidneys are the first to be observed in people with diabetes.

Sushruta was also aware of the structures of the heart and its role in the circulation of 'vital fluids' through the 'channels', and gave accounts of angina—chest pain on exertion, and high blood pressure (Dwivedi and Chaturvedi 2000). Without available drugs, Sushruta treated diabetes, angina and atherosclerosis (fatty deposits in the arteries) with plant medicine (Kansupada and Sassani 1997). In ancient times, atherosclerosis was common. When scanned, ancient mummies have shown this to be the case in preindustrial civilisations, suggesting that some people had a tendency towards this particular condition.

Surgery was very advanced in ancient India. Injury and disease often led to amputation, although Indian physicians had minimal knowledge of anatomy due to religious beliefs making internal investigation of the human body forbidden. It is probable that patients with diabetes would be among those requiring limb amputation. If the patient survived the surgery, infection often killed, as high blood glucose levels would not have helped healing.

Today, other than the result of an accident, diabetes is the most common cause of amputation, with lower limb amputations being 15–40 times more likely in those with diabetes (van Dieren et al. 2010).

Ancient Egypt

Ancient Egyptian medicine was a refined balance of practical knowledge and religious beliefs. While they used natural remedies and surgical techniques, they also incorporated magic and incantations into their healing practices.

Understanding of anatomy and disease was relatively advanced for the time, with knowledge documented through various papyri, which are still studied today. The Egyptian Empire acquired medical knowledge through conquest, and it is recorded that one of the first texts mentioning symptoms similar to diabetes was *The Ebers Papyrus*.

Egyptian physician, *Hesy-Ra*, of the Third Dynasty in 1536 B.C. felt that symptoms—such as raging thirst and frequent urination—were unusual and important enough to document. The discovery of a medical papyrus between the legs of a mummy in Thebes heralded the first description of diabetes. In an excellent state of preservation and reportedly wrapped in mummy cloths, the text was written in hieratic, a form of hieroglyphic writing used by priests, with 877 section headings, finishing with a calendar which allowed it to be dated to the ninth year of the reign of Amenophis in 1536 B.C. (Ghalioungui 1987).

The scroll's content suggests that the papyrus was a summary of knowledge drawn from a number of books many centuries older, with one passage dating from the First Dynasty B.C. (circa 3400). German Egyptologist, Georg Ebers was first shown this perfectly preserved papyrus in 1872 and he immediately raised the money to purchase it, donating the find—named *The Ebers Papyrus* in his honour—to the library at the University of Leipzig (Bryan 1974).

The Ebers Papyrus is considered the most complete surviving ancient Egyptian medical text (Bryan 1974). The scroll contains magical formulas and folk remedies meant to cure a number of afflictions ranging from crocodile bites to toenail pain, and to rid the house of such pests as flies, rats and scorpions. The *Ebers Papyrus* is reportedly one of the oldest medical texts known to man, dating from the second millennium B.C.

Ebers produced the entire manuscript shortly afterwards, with the help of his colleague, Ludwig Stern. Four English translations were later produced in the twentieth century, the last being the most comprehensive, although both hieratic and hieroglyphic texts were not included (Ghalioungui 1987).

Treatments

The Ebers Papyrus refers to kidney and urinary conditions. Ancient Egyptian physicians did not understand that diabetes was a specific disease, but they did recognise the symptoms of frequent urination and thirst. As can be seen below, many of the remedies appear to address the same symptoms; remedies are given in *The Ebers Papyrus* for (Loriaux 2006):

- The passing of large quantities of urine
- Correcting urine that is in excess
- Correcting the urine of a child
- The child suffering from urinary incontinence
- Reduction of the urine when it is too plentiful
- Controlling fast-flowing urine
- Collecting urine together to concentrate it and decrease the flow
- For collecting the urine in the diseased pubic region at the first occurrence of suffering

Before the discovery of insulin, people with type 1 diabetes became very thin because insulin helps the body use glucose for fuel. Without enough insulin, the body turns to burning fat and muscle as an energy source. Only one section of *The Ebers Papyrus* seems to mention emaciation of a person with untreated type 1 diabetes mellitus (Bryan 1974):

> If you examine someone sick [within] the centre of his being [digestive organs] [and] if his body is shrunken with disease at its limit; if you examine him [and] you do not find disease in [his] body except for the surface of the ribs [emaciation] of which members [stick out] you should then [a spell to remedy] disease this in your house; you should then prepare for him ingredients for [treating] it; ground blood stone; red grain; carob; cook in oil [and] honey; [it] should be eaten by him over mornings four for the suppression of his thirst [and] for curing his mortal illness.

The causes of disease were mysterious in ancient Egypt, attributable to magic and curses. Many Egyptians believed in the power of unfriendly magic, along with evil spirits as a cause of disease. Without a knowledge of the disease process, fear and retribution prevailed, rather than looking for the reason for illness (Nutton 2005).

People with visible disease have always been shunned by society. A debilitating physical or mental disorder was solid proof of spiritual corruption of the body, where disease originated from sin. With its magical and religious connotations, there was a great fear of disease; it was believed that the affliction, whatever its symptoms, could be passed on to others in close proximity to the person who was unwell.

This reaction is fully justified with a contagious infection like the flu or tuberculosis, although the core belief at the time was that to stay healthy, the spirits should not be angered, unfortunately meaning individuals with debilitating diseases were punished for their sins. Displeasing the gods was also believed to result in evil spirits and their poisons, necessitating the cleansing of the body with prayers, incantations and the injection of various concoctions into the orifices of the body (Nunn 1996).

As the causes of disease were not understood, the use of magic and observation was the only treatment. Even today, sympathetic magic is believed to work on similarity. Ancient Egyptian medicine therefore held that disease could be healed if an object possessed certain qualities, repelling the source of evil by creating a sympathetic action in the form of incantations and actions.

From as early as the fifth century B.C. the Egyptians understood that certain diseases required the specialist knowledge of a medical consultant (Zucconi 2007). A patient with the symptoms of diabetes may well have visited an expert in urinary complaints in order to find a remedy for excessive urinary flow, unstoppable thirst, weight loss and weakness. *Herodotus*, The Greek historian and traveller, wrote about the types of medical practitioners in Egypt (Strassler and Purvis 2008):

> The art of healing is with them divided up, so that each physician treats one ailment and no more. Egypt is full of physicians, some treating diseases in the eyes, others the head, others the teeth, others the stomach and others unspecified disease.

Physicians in fifth-century Egypt had only modest anatomical knowledge, and did not prepare bodies for the mummification process, which would have led to a far greater understanding (Nutton 2005). It was not until around 350 B.C. with the work of *Herophilus* and *Eristratus* that a basic knowledge of the connection between the pulse and the heart reached ancient Greece. Anatomists were then able to advance their knowledge of the human body to include the bones and limbs following observations made during severe injury.

Dissection of the human body went against religious beliefs; this practice did not form a vital part of medical education until the mid-sixteenth century; animal dissections were the only way to advance understanding of structures and systems, allowing assumptions to be drawn about similarities in human anatomy, although these were often incorrect (Nutton 2005).

Early Treatments

As we have seen, *The Ebers Papyrus* suggests healing preparations for some main symptoms of diabetes, a disorder considered to originate in the urinary tract or kidneys because of the development of excessive thirst and frequent urination (Loriaux 2006). From the modern standpoint of understanding, it is concerning that ancient Egyptian physicians frequently prescribed honey or sweet beer for urinary incontinence and great thirst (Bryan 1974).

Dates (the fruit of the date palm) were also added to three of the treatments documented in *The Ebers Papyrus* for urinary overflow, dates also being a favourite laxative (Georgacarakos 2011). Honey had a therapeutic use in treating illness, and today we recognise that honey boosts the immune system. We now know that treatments containing honey would have hastened a patient's death without insulin to treat them.

Glucose thickens the blood, making the heart work much harder. This leads to enlargement of the heart and eventual heart disease, ultimately resulting in an early death.

Egyptian physicians tried to balance the patient's body fluids by putting sweetness back into the body to compensate for urinary loss. Excessive urination in diabetes is due to an abnormal amount of glucose in the blood which the kidneys try to excrete from the body. This causes the patient to lose a great deal of fluid, and they are forced to drink excessively to readjust their fluid balance.

According to *The Ebers Papyrus*, frequent urination and intense thirst were additionally managed with herbal, plant and natural medicines (Loriaux 2006) which we recognise today as having a moderate effect on reducing glucose levels. Patients would be told to eat onions and garlic frequently, containing compounds of sulphur which have blood glucose lowering properties (Sheela and Augusti 1992). Coriander seeds and leaves were also used for various urinary complaints (Murray 1995).

These remedies suggest that physicians were aware of the need to reduce glucose and treat frequent urination. *The Ebers Papyrus* also documents the use of copper compounds for growths in the neck—which were possibly boils—and itching (Dollwet and Sorenson 1985): two further symptoms of excessive glucose in the body. The need for a balanced diet was also recognised by Egyptian physicians. Ancient Egyptians ate a diet containing carbohydrates from cereals, proteins (mostly from fish), and fruits and vegetables; milk products, seeds and oils were consumed less often (Zucconi 2007). Eating a balanced diet is recommended for everyone today, including those with diabetes mellitus.

Interpretation

As we can see, ancient Egyptian physicians appear to have been aware of excess sugar as the cause of frequent urination in their patients. The use of a type of homeopathic remedy to replace sweetness that was lost is extremely forward-thinking, if incorrect. There are numerous recipes for urinary complaints, but as diabetes was not recognised as a condition in its own right, these recipes were not used for the treatment of diabetes.

Other conditions of the bladder could be aggravated by the use of sweet recipes, and in themselves result in more frequent urination. Although not linked to diabetes, conditions such as cystitis—inflammation of the bladder—would have been worsened by an intake of sugary fluids as sugar exacerbates inflammation.

A far rarer type of diabetes is diabetes insipidus. This condition is characterised by large amounts of dilute urine and increased thirst. The amount of urine produced can be as much as 20 litres per day. Reduction of fluid has little effect on the concentration of the urine. What makes diabetes insipidus different from diabetes mellitus is that there is no excretion of glucose in the urine.

Prehistoric dental records show that health was poor in ancient civilisations, with widespread malnutrition and, if depictions of the ancient Egyptians serve as a guideline, obesity was not common (Bryan 1974). Consequently, obesity associated with type 2 diabetes was rarely seen. Egyptian physicians would only have infrequently encountered patients with childhood type 1 diabetes, or the far rarer diabetes insipidus.

Ancient Persia

As medical wisdom spread across civilisations, the skills and knowledge of ancient Persian physicians became heavily influenced by other growing cultures and their advances in medicine. Persian interest in Greek medicine was seen when *Hippocrates* (circa 460–370 B.C.) was asked by the King of Persia to use his extensive medical knowledge to help with the epidemics and diseases afflicting his people (Schneider and Lilienfeld 2008).

Early Treatments

As in each ancient civilisation, diabetes in Persia was treated using herbs and plant extracts, such as wild rue, barsam—possibly balsam pear, known for its glucose-reducing effects, extracts from mint (Mentha spicata) and Egyptian willow, as well as concoctions made from multiple herbs (*Cambridge Illustrated History of Medicine* 2001). Writing a number of medical books, Erasistratus championed the use of a modest diet to cure diseases such as diabetes over the use of herbs or bloodletting to reduce the symptoms (Wootton 2006; Nutton 2005). This approach is key for treating type 2 diabetes today.

In ancient Iran, the earliest available medical text was the *Avesta*—a collection of religious writings compiled around the sixth century B.C., although the exact date is unknown (Georgacarakos 2011). Of the four surviving texts of the *Avesta*, the *Videvdat* describes the required education and experience of physicians, magic and herbal remedies, and surgical techniques. Book four, the *Gyaah Pezeshk* (herbal medicine) documents the importance of herbal remedies (Darmester 1898):

> We worship all herbs, we seek them, we hold them in awe in order to fight death and sickness. (Chapter 20, verse 6)

Religious beliefs dictated that disease was the result of failing to worship the gods correctly. In order to appease them, healthcare in ancient times was provided in temples named after the gods. In common with ancient Greece, patients did not actually stay in these temples during the duration of their illness to receive treatment and recuperate; healing temples were places used only for the diagnosis of illness to find the cause, much like a modern doctor's surgery (Elgood 1951). Diagnosis of disease was often assisted by up-to-date medical texts. Most healthcare needs were treated in the home, though some religious healing ceremonies believed that river waters would wash away the evil sources of disease (Gorji and Ghadiri 2006).

Alexander the Great encouraged the assimilation of Hellenic (Greek) thinking, including their not inconsiderable medical knowledge, into Persian tradition; with this knowledge, Greek medical texts were translated into Persian and then Arabic (Georgacarakos 2011). The city of Alexandria became part of Egypt when Alexander the Great conquered Egypt in 332 B.C. The city of Alexandria in the fourth century B.C. was at the forefront of medical knowledge. The completion of the Alexandrian library and museum in 275 B.C. attracted scholars to what was to become a renowned medical research institution (Georgacarakos 2011).

Important advances in anatomical knowledge of the brain and nervous system were made during this period; these are attributable to two eminent Persian physicians, *Herophilos of Chalcedon* and *Erasistratus of Ioulis* (von Straden 2007). Ancient civilisations gained considerable anatomical knowledge from the battlefield. With the relaxation of dissection laws, progress was made in the field of human anatomy. It is possible that Herophilus practised his dissection techniques on deceased criminals in order to establish the anatomy of the brain and its relationship to the nerves; following the period of Herophilus and Eristratus, however, vivisection and dissection ceased for several hundred years (Wootton 2006).

What of Diabetes?

It was the valuable work of Herophilos that led to medical advancements; especially important was recognising the diagnostic value of the pulse as an indicator of ill health (Gorji and Ghadiri 2006). Herophilos considered that the symptoms of diabetes were a kind of *dropsy*—fluid accumulation in the body cavities (Peitzman 2008), now known as congestive heart disease. It is clearly seen that at this time, diabetes was regarded as a kidney disease with the only remedies being herbal medicine.

In common with ancient Egypt, Persian physicians attributed the root of disease to antagonised spirits, ghosts or the wrath of the gods; each spirit was held responsible for bringing about a specific disease (Nutton 2005). One feared spirit was Lamashtu, she-demon of disease and death; it was widely believed that her wrath caused organs of the body to suddenly malfunction, bringing disease (Elgood 1951).

The practice of dissection allowed the examination of human organs, a key advancement on using animals to gain anatomical knowledge. Herophilos described the pancreas as an important organ in 300 B.C., although it took a further 2000 years for destruction of the insulin-producing cells of the pancreas to be associated with type 1 diabetes (von Straden 2007). In the fourth century B.C., the diagnosis of disease, including diabetes, was accomplished with the observation of urine, sputum, saliva and the pulse (Nutton 2005).

Understanding Diabetes

The majority of medical knowledge in this era was based on the Avestan sciences (Gorji and Ghadiri 2006; Elgood 1951). The practice of medicine and education in this area were highly valued, as was the need to bring together available medical knowledge, thinking and practices to treat disease. In this way, the examination by observation of urine became a highly advanced practice (Gorji and Ghadiri 2006). Medical knowledge regarding diabetes was greatly enhanced by Persian scientists; their in-depth observations would later become the science of endocrinology.

Due to ancient Iran's chaotic history, many prestigious medical libraries and millions of books containing the wisdom of the ancients were unfortunately destroyed, including some very valuable medical texts (Nutton 2005). As a result, remaining ancient Egyptian documentation of medical practices and texts brought about the most enduring influence through spreading medical knowledge and practices via the ancient Greeks (*Cambridge Illustrated History of Medicine* 2001).

From 750–900 A.D. the chief Muslim and political rulers (Caliphs) demanded that books be acquired from Greece, India and Egypt among others, especially in the fields of medicine, astronomy and mathematics; these included texts from their enemies (Durant 1950). A scientific college, observatory and public library were established by 830 A.D. where predominantly ancient Greek and Indian scholarly texts were translated into Arabic, notably preserving over a hundred medical treatises by the Greek physician, *Galen*. Bringing together ancient knowledge in these areas was a huge task, but by 850 A.D., most of the classical Greek and Hindu texts had been translated (Durant 1950).

Ancient Greece

Greek physicians were influenced by contemporary cultures. They too explored how diseases developed, forming their own treatments and diagnostic methods. Around 450 B.C., the Greek philosopher and physician, *Alcmaeon* was the first to suggest that disease originated from opposing factors such as heat and cold, or wetness and dryness, creating an imbalance (Miller et al. 2010a).

This theory was expanded by Hippocrates (circa 460–370 B.C.), known as 'the father of medicine', who completely disregarded supernatural causes of disease. Retaining the theory of imbalance as the root of all disease, he proposed that health was achieved with a balance in the four bodily 'humours'. Hippocrates drew this theory from the four natural elements of Greek physics: earth, water, air and fire (Schneider and Lilienfeld 2008).

The four humours of the body—blood, phlegm, yellow bile and black bile—were believed to be linked to the four major organs: the heart, the brain, the liver and the spleen. Hippocrates believed that it was important to keep a balance between all four humours for health, and any imbalance would need to be rectified. This belief in humoural balance was recorded in the first century, after Hippocrates' lifetime. Treatments to restore humoural balance included bloodletting by cutting a vein, and by applying leeches; the use of emetics—substances to induce vomiting, and purgatives; and cautery using hot irons applied to various parts of the body (Wootton 2006). Ironically, most of these treatments were detrimental to health.

Diabetes in Ancient Greece

Apollonius of Memphis described the severe symptoms of the sufferer, naming the disease 'diabetes', the Ionian Greek for siphon in 230 B.C. Hippocrates believed that experiment and observation to gain experience were the only true methods to discover the causes of disease. In common with modern thinking about diabetes, he advocated that although it was possible to overcome illness, the correct diet enabled a balance to be achieved in the body fluids. In his medical writings he mentions the most prominent symptoms of type 1 diabetes: excessive urinary flow, and a wasting disease of the body (Schneider and Lilienfeld 2008).

Regular exercise and a moderate lifestyle in conjunction with a good diet encourage the absence of disease. The mainstay of staying well with diabetes today, this was advised by Hippocrates in the fifth century B.C. Despite this clear awareness of preventing obesity and type 2 diabetes, Hippocrates did not suggest any specific treatment for diabetes itself. This is perhaps because Hippocrates and his followers believed that medicine did not offer any useful benefit for internal conditions like diabetes (Wootton 2006).

The observations of Hippocrates on diet are similar to those of the Greek philosopher, *Plato*, (circa 428–343 B.C.), who also favoured a moderate intake of cereals, milk, honey, fish and fruit, with wine, meat and confectionary only eaten occasionally (Nutton 2005). In Plato's opinion, excesses of food resulted in ill health—a very astute observation. This could be viewed as a warning that without moderation, obesity occurs, which can lead to type 2 diabetes.

Symptoms

In 250 B.C., the Greek physician *Arateus* described diabetes as 'the melting down of flesh and limbs into urine' (Reed 1954). This very accurate image exactly captures the symptoms of severe insulin deficiency—known medically as *hyperglycaemia* and *ketoacidosis*.

Hyperglycaemia describes the high concentration of glucose in the blood in the absence of insulin to help the use of glucose as energy. Ketoacidosis describes the breakdown of fats and muscle for fuel when glucose levels are high.

Galen, writing over 400 years later in 180 A.D., observed type 1 diabetes to be very rare (Johnston 2006). Describing and discussing diabetes in a number of his works, Galen writes that the condition was seldom seen on the basis that he had only encountered two cases in his medical career (Johnston 2006). This suggests he saw cases of the less-common type 1 diabetes, or perhaps two patients with the even rarer condition, diabetes insipidus.

Galen describes the symptoms he observed in these patients as 'diarrhoea urinosa'—an outpouring of urine, and 'dipsakos'—the thirsty disease, which he used in his writings when referring to the condition of diabetes. Due to the prominence of frequent urination, Galen believed diabetes to be a disease of the kidneys. Although he understood kidney function, he was unaware of their position in the human body; writing on the subject of diabetes in his book, *On the Localisation of Diseases*, Galen states (Johnston 2006):

> I am of the opinion that the kidneys too are affected in the rare disease that some people call chamber-pot dropsy, others again diabetes or violent thirst. For my own part I have seen the disease till now only twice when the patient suffered from an inextinguishable thirst, which forced them to drink enormous quantities; the fluid was urinated swiftly with a urine resembling the drink.

The above passage describes the patient's urine being so dilute with all the fluid taken in that it resembled water when it was passed out of the body. Galen categorised the condition of diabetes as a 'genuine kidney disease, analogous to a voracious appetite' (Johnston 2006).

Untreated type 1 diabetes does not allow glucose to be used by the cells of the body. When the patient eats, carbohydrate is broken down into glucose, although this cannot enter the cells without sufficient insulin.

The word 'diabetes' was already in common usage in Galen's time, although accounts differ over who was the first to use the term in their writing. It is believed that 'diabetes' was commonly understood by early physicians, although it is not known exactly from where the term originated. There are differing accounts concerning when the term came into use: the term 'diabetes' has been attributed to both Aretaeus of Cappodocia, a follower of Hippocrates in the second century A.D., and *Apollonius of Memphis* in 230 B.C. (Reed 1954).

Aretaeus of Cappodocia gave an account of the chronic and devastating nature of type 1 diabetes, naming it the Greek word 'diabaino', meaning 'go' or 'run through', and 'diabetes' meaning siphon or water pipe (translated by Adams 1856):

> For the fluids do not remain in the body, but use the body only as a channel through which they flow out. Life lasts only for a time, but not very long. For they urinate with pain and painful is the emaciation. For no essential part of the drink is absorbed by the body while great masses of the flesh are liquefied into urine.

Aretaeus of Cappodocia described the onset of type 1 diabetes in the following way: 'great masses of flesh are liquefied into urine'. This is very similar to the account of diabetes given by the earlier Aretaeus in 250 B.C., around 300 years previously: 'the melting down of flesh and limbs into urine'. It is highly possible that Aretaeus of Cappodocia had read the earlier account before giving his own similar description.

There are no existing records documenting the occurrence and frequency of cases of diabetes across ancient Greece. Observing that the affliction of diabetes 'is not very frequent among men' (Reed 1954), Aretaeus of Cappodocia was perhaps observing that the condition was more common in the female population of Greece. This suggests the onset of gestational diabetes in pregnancy, or that it was simply not a common disease.

Gestational diabetes occurs when a hormone made by the placenta prevents the body from using insulin effectively, causing glucose to build up in the blood instead of being absorbed by the cells.

As we have seen, Galen—writing 400 years after Aretaeus of Cappodocia—also described diabetes as very rare. The type of diabetes being described in the writings of both physicians is unclear, although the rarity of the condition is emphasised (Johnston 2006). This may suggest that type 2 diabetes would be seen more often, given its association with obesity, an inactive lifestyle and the inability of insulin to work well in the presence of excess body fat.

The symptoms described in the following account (Reed 1954) could equally refer to either type 1 or type 2 diabetes (translated by Adams 1856):

> The patient never stops making water, but the flow is incessant, as if from the opening of aqueducts [applicable to type 1]. The nature of the disease, then, is chronic, and it takes a long period to form [distinctive of type 2]: but the patient is short-lived [describing untreated type 1]. If the constitution of the disease be completely established, the melting is rapid, the death speedy [type 1].

Aretaeus of Cappodocia went on to describe an unquenchable, burning thirst—known medically as *polydipsia*—which, if the patient did not take a drink, resulted in a parched mouth and nausea, followed by death (Reed 1954). This is undoubtedly a description of untreated type 1 diabetes. The Greek physician likened the thirst to being (translated by Adams 1856):

> Scorched up with fire, although the patient's temperature is not high, they experience a burning sensation seated in the intestines [acidity in type 1 diabetes?] The abdomen becomes shrivelled and the veins protuberant [severe dehydration in untreated type 1], with a sensitivity at the extremity of the member before making more urine.

Aretaeus of Cappodocia also noted that 'many parts of the flesh pass out with the urine' (Reed 1954). This conclusion would have been based on observation alone, as the ancient Greeks had no means of chemically testing the urine. With our modern understanding of what happens in untreated diabetes, we know that a lack of insulin leads to the breakdown of fats into ketone bodies that are present with high blood glucose levels. However, it appears that 'great masses of flesh liquefied into urine' (Aretaeus of Cappodocia) and the earlier but similar, 'the melting down of flesh and limbs into urine' (Arateus), describe this process. This no doubt refers to extreme weight loss in untreated type 1 diabetes.

In his book, *Therapeutics of Chronic Disease*, Aretaeus of Cappodocia provides his explanation of the disease process in diabetes, likening its symptoms to those of dropsy (Reed 1954), where excess fluid accumulates in the body cavities (translated by Adams 1856):

> The flow of humour from the affected part of the melting is the same [as in dropsy], but the defluxation [outpouring] is determined to the kidneys and bladder. In diabetes the thirst is greater for the fluid running off dries the body. For the thirst there is need of a powerful remedy, for in kind it is the greatest of all sufferings; and when a fluid is drunk it stimulates discharge of urine.

Again, this describes untreated type 1 diabetes. Type 2 diabetes has a much slower onset, with noticeable symptoms not always present. Patients without urgent symptoms needing a doctor's attention may therefore have gone undocumented in ancient Greece.

> We now know that type 2 diabetes can be present as prediabetes with raised glucose levels, but no significant symptoms for 10–15 years before diagnosis during a routine blood test (Sagesaka et al. 2018).

Treatments

Drug remedies for disease, including diabetes, were not widely available as the science of chemistry was not yet a standard practice (Nutton 2005). Physicians prescribed various ingredients in their concoctions to treat ailments and it would be hard to identify between the active ingredients of these when taken as a remedy. It was not until the end of the Hellenic period (31 B.C.) and the beginning of the classical period in the sixth to fourth centuries B.C. that treatments for ill health were managed using a prescription format (Nutton 2005), formulating medical practices.

Literary texts and archaeological records show that ancient Greek physicians had knowledge of many remedies (pharmacea) from plants, herbs, animals, metals and minerals (Nutton 2005). Galen (circa 128–201 A.D.) and Aretaeus of Cappodocia (second century A.D.) followed the teachings of Hippocrates; Galen recommended a diet of fish, fowl, barley, beans, onions and garlic to 'thin the humours' of patients with chronic (long-standing) disease, while bloodletting was seen as an extension of dietary therapy because it restored the balance of an unhealthy diet (Wootton 2006). As a treatment for diabetes, Aretaeus of Cappodocia prescribed oil of roses, dates, raw quinces and gruel (Reed 1954). As with ancient Egyptian treatments, dates appear in the recipe, possibly to act as a laxative to flush the disease.

In 55 A.D., *Pedianos Dioscorides* (father of pharmacology) wrote his *De Materia Medica* (Castleden 1994), listing 1000 unmixed remedies. The word 'medicine', meaning drug, comes from his *Materia Medica* (Wootton 2006).

People with type 2 diabetes of a longer duration (a few years) would most probably have developed secondary health issues, like cataracts, due to persistently high glucose levels. The *Materia Medica* shows how to produce verdigris by exposing metallic copper to boiling vinegar, providing blue-green copper acetate as a remedy for cataract, amongst other ailments, given in the form of eye drops known as *collyria* (Dollwet and Sorenson 1985).

Ancient Rome

Ancient Rome had assimilated the medical ideas of the Egyptians and Greeks, so there was no new perspective on health and illness. Diabetes was viewed as a disease of the kidneys because of the excessive thirst and urination accompanying the untreated condition. It was only later in classical Greece (550–300 B.C.) that physicians such as Hippocrates suggested that diseases like diabetes were due to an abnormality of the humours, rather than a punishment by the gods.

Many Greek physicians migrated to Rome after the Romans conquered the Macedonians in 197 B.C. These medical specialists included Galen as physician to the court of Emperor Marcus Aurelius and three of his successors (Johnston 2006). Combining Greek medical thinking with Roman medicine was not readily accepted; it seemed to some that doctors might be trying to charge rich patients a large fee for their medicines in order to make money, rather than to enable recovery. Gargilius Martialis wrote (Johnston 2006):

> Some doctors charge the most excessive prices for the most worthless medicines and drugs, and others in the craft attempt to deal with and treat diseases they obviously do not understand.

In his book, *On Natural History*, *Pliny the Elder* (23–79 A.D.) recorded that the first doctor (medicus) invited to visit Rome from Greece was *Archagathus* in 291 B.C. (Pliny the Elder and Healey 1991), although doctors then were not the educated, skilled professionals they are today.

In his treatise *On Natural History*, Pliny the Elder observed: ‘Garlic has powerful properties and provides defence during changes of water’ (Pliny the Elder and Healey 1991). Garlic and onions were often used as a stomach remedy by the Egyptians, but were also thought to reduce the severity of diabetes symptoms when frequently consumed. Today we know that onions and garlic contain sulphur compounds that have minimal blood glucose-lowering effects.

Poor knowledge of the causes and spread of disease meant recovery from any illness was not straightforward. In the second century B.C. Roman medicine centred around agriculture and simple remedies for ill health taken at home (*Cambridge Illustrated History of Medicine* 2001). Many diseases had obscure treatments, such as wool, and the power of cabbages, according to Pliny the Elder and *Cato the Elder* (Pliny the Elder and Healey 1991; Miller et al. 2010b).

Galen wrote on the production of urine in his book *On the Natural Faculties*. His knowledge was determined via experimentation with animals to gain insight into diseases that alter kidney function, like diabetes (Galen et al. 2011).

Galen and his students had focused their work around the bodies of Barbary apes and pigs instead of human bodies. As an anatomist, Galen believed the pancreas protected the stomach and other vessels in the abdomen (Galen et al. 2011). For centuries, this view remained unchallenged. Progressive anatomical and physiological research slowed dramatically after Galen's death in 201 A.D. in the belief that the prominent physician had already explored every aspect of medicine so extensively.

Accepted without question, Galen's theories on disease and medical practices were considered the very best available; Roman religious beliefs forbade human dissection, meaning his ideas went unchallenged. It was not until 1543 B.C. that *Vesalius* drew attention to over 300 anatomical mistakes, where Galen had drawn his conclusions on human anatomy from the dissection of animals.

In *De Medicina* (circa 40 A.D.) *Aulus Cornelius Celsus* wrote that the Art of Medicine was threefold: cure through diet; cure through medicaments—not purgatives and emetics, but oils, poultices, embrocations and liniments applied to the outside of the body, and cure 'by hand', meaning surgery. Celsus identified three types of practitioners (Wootton 2006):

- Dogmatists—followers of Herophilus, who believed in finding hidden causes to explain biological processes (believers in vivisection and dissection).
- Methodists, who could be trained in 6 months—gave a simple mechanical explanation for disease being due to particles travelling either too fast or too slowly through the body.
- Empirics, believing that all theories of disease must be rejected, relying on experience to know which interventions were effective (Wootton 2006).

Complications of Diabetes

Although a degree of quackery was involved in medicine, importance was placed on surgical and clinical care to treat eye disease, with texts suggesting that this knowledge went back much further (*Cambridge Illustrated History of Medicine* 2001).

Celsus classed diabetes mellitus as a 'disease of excess urination and wasting' (Miller et al. 2010a), using the patient's urine as a diagnostic tool. He understood that diabetes was associated with other health complaints (complications). Celsus would treat cataracts using specific eye surgery, known as couching, where the lens of the eye is moved out of the line of sight using a needle to cut if free. Without a lens the patient's vision would be blurry, only seeing colours and vague shapes rather than any detail, such as being able to read.

With consistently high blood glucose levels, nerve damage and impaired blood circulation, skin ulceration of the lower limbs was a common problem. For non-healing chronic ulceration of the skin on the legs or feet, Celsus recommended a balm containing copper oxide applied to the skin (Dollwet and Sorenson 1985). Even today, one of the main complications of poor circulation and slow healing in diabetes is foot and leg ulcers.

The Pancreas

Rufus of Ephesus was a Greco-Roman physician and anatomist. He recognised the importance of the pancreas in 100 A.D., giving the organ its name meaning 'pan'—all, and 'creas'—flesh. He discovered that the organ 'was not soft, had a similar consistency throughout and did not contain any bones' (Eknoyan 2002).

At the end of the first century A.D., Rufus of Ephesus wrote the first book dedicated to diseases of the kidneys and bladder, examining the composition and purpose of the kidneys, observing how disease affects these organs (Eknoyan 2002).

Chronic changes in kidney tissue occur due to continually high blood glucose levels. Rufus of Ephesus observed this in part of his work, describing hardening and stiffening of the kidney tissues. We know today that if unchecked, this deterioration leads to kidney failure.

The Romans finally withdrew from Britain from 407 A.D., heralding a slow demise of Roman influence (Castleden 1994). When the Romans left Britain they took their medical knowledge with them, halting any new research. With the Saxon invasion around 449 A.D., there began the Great Exodus of Romanised Britains from England, who took Christianity, literacy and practical knowledge with them. Ireland saw the increase of Christianity, the number of monasteries, hospitals and libraries; without these monasteries, culture, learning and writing would have been eradicated from Western Europe (Castleden 1994). The continuing power of the written word preserved ancient knowledge for future generations.

After the fall of the Roman Empire in the fifth century A.D., important medical texts, including those of Galen, were lost, although many were later rediscovered in the libraries of the Moorish Empire (modern-day Spain, Portugal and North Africa), having a profound influence on European medical practices (Green 2007).

Summary

Through conflict and the establishment of trade routes, the spread of medical knowledge and of new ideas into the ancient civilisations of China, India, Egypt, Persia, Greece and Rome, shaped the basis of medicine and its practice. Type 1 diabetes was thought of as a rapid wasting disease and a death sentence, which could not be effectively eased with herbal and plant remedies in the absence of insulin.

Type 2 diabetes, where dietary changes and herbal remedies were partially effective, was observed to be more common among the richer classes in the presence of obesity and an inactive lifestyle. Today people with type 2 diabetes take insulin when glucose-reducing drugs fail to work effectively after several years. Type 2 diabetes was often successfully treated with a change in lifestyle, adopting a moderate diet and introducing regular exercise into the routine. This approach is still favoured today, although without glucose-reducing medicines, diabetes patients in the ancient world would have faced a much shorter lifespan.

Certain herbs and plants were used for their recognised glucose-reducing effects when eaten regularly. Physicians were aware that the high levels of 'sugar' in patients with diabetes was making them ill, although this could not be effectively tested. It was not known why this disease resulted in high sugar levels, although some of the chronic long-term complications of diabetes were recognised as due to the primary condition. These secondary conditions were treated with early medicine, such as the surgical extraction of cataracts in ancient India and Rome.

Diabetes in ancient times was viewed as a disease affecting both the kidneys and the bladder because of its hallmark symptoms of excessive thirst and frequent urination. This thinking was to last for more than 2000 years.

References

Adams F (1856) Aretaeus (1856). The extant works, Edited and translated by Francis Adams. Royal Society (reprint), Milford House Inc, London/Boston. 1972

Bridgewater NJ (2001) Historical aspects of diabetic neuropathies. In: Ward JD (ed) Diabetic neuropathy. Royal Society of Chemistry/Aventis, London, pp 6–15

Bryan CP (ed) (1974) Ancient Egyptian medicine: the papyrus Ebers. Ares, Chicago

Cambridge Illustrated History of Medicine (2001) History of disease. London: Cambridge University Press, 16–51

Castleden R (1994) World history: a chronological history of dates. Parragon Book Service Limited, London

Darmester J (1898) AVESTA: VENDIDAD: the origins of medicine, Translated from sacred books of the east American Edition. The Christian Literature Company, New York

Dharmananda S (2002) Treatment of diabetes with Chinese herbs and acupuncture. Internet Journal of the Institute for Traditional Medicine and Preventative Healthcare http://www.itmonline.org/journal/arts/diabetes.htm

Dollwet HHA, Sorenson JRJ (1985) Historic uses of copper compounds in medicine. Trace Elem Med 2(2):80–87

Durant W (1950) Age of faith (the story of civilization). In: The story of civilization Part IV. The Book Service, Colchester, Essex, pp 162–186

Dwivedi S, Chaturvedi A (2000) Cardiology in ancient India. J Indian Coll Cardiol 1:8–15

Dwivedi G, Dwivedi S (2007) Sushruta—the clinician—teacher par excellence. Indian J Chest Dis Allied Sci 49:243–244

Eknoyan G (2002) Rufus of Ephesus and his diseases of the kidney. Nephron 91(3):383–390

Elgood C (1951) A medical history of Persia and the eastern caliphate from the earliest times to the year 1932 AD. Cambridge University Press, London, pp 205–209

Frank LL (1957) Diabetes mellitus in the texts of old Hindu medicine. Am J Gastroenterol 27:76

Galen, Horsley GHR, Johnston I (eds) (2011) Method of medicine: books 1–4. The Maple-Vail Book Manufacturing Group, New York

Gearson S (1993) Ayurveda: the ancient Indian healing art. Element Books, Shaftsbury

Georgacarakos M (2011) Ancient traditional medicine of Byzantine, Egypt, Greece, Medieval, Islam, Iran, and Rome. Lightening Source UK, Milton Keynes

Ghalioungui P (1987) The Ebers Papyrus: a new English translation, commentaries, and glossaries. Academy of Scientific Research and Technology, Cairo

Gorji A, Ghadiri MK (2006) Contributions of Iranian scientists to medicine: ancient and medieval periods. Kanun Med J 8:xx–xxx

Green P (2007) Alexander the Great and the Hellenistic age: a short history (universal history). Weidenfeld and Nicholson, London

Hikino H (1991) Traditional remedies and modern assessment; the case of ginseng. In: Wijeskera ROB (ed) The medical plant industry. CRC Press, Boca Raton, pp 149–166

Holmes P (1997) Jade remedies: a Chinese herbal reference for the West. University of Minnesota Press: Snow Lotus Productions

Hong-Yen H, Peacher WG (1978) Chen's history of Chinese medical science. Oriental Healing Arts Institute, Long Beach

Johnston I (2006) Galen: on diseases and symptoms. Cambridge University Press, London, pp 50–72

Kansupada KB, Sassani JW (1997) Sushruta, the father of Indian surgery and ophthalmology. Doc Ophthalmol 93:159–167

Kutumbian P (2005) Ancient Indian medicine. Orient Longman, Hyderabad; reprinted edition

Loriaux DL (2006) The Ebers Papyrus 1552 B.C. Endocrinologist 16(2):55–56

Maoshing N (1995) The yellow emperor's classic of medicine: a new translation of the Neijing Suwen with commentary. Shambhala, Boston

Miller FM, Vandrome AF, McBrewster J (eds) (2010a) Aulus Cornelius Celsus: De Medicina, Praenomen, Augustus, Tiberius, Themison of Laodicea, Gallia Narbonesis, Pliny the Elder, Quintilian, Hippocrates, Columella. Alphascript Publishing, Beau Basin

Miller FM, Vandrome AF, McBrewster J (eds) (2010b) Cato the Elder. Alphascript Publishing, Beau Bassin

Mukherjee PK, Kuntal M, Kakali M et al (2006) Leads from Indian medicinal plants with hypoglycaemic potentials. J Ethnopharmacol 106(1):1–28

Murray MT (1995) The healing power of herbs, 2nd edn. Gramercy Books, New York, pp 265–271

Nadkarmi KM (2005) The Indian Materia Medica. Volume II. Popular Prakashan Limited, Mumbai, pp 23–32

Ng TB, Yeung HW (1982) Hypoglycaemic constituents of *Panax* ginseng. Gen Pharmacol 6:549–552

Nunn JF (1996) Ancient Egyptian medicine. University of Oklahoma Press, Norman

Nutton V (2005) Ancient medicine (science of antiquity series). Routledge, Taylor and Francis Group, London

Peitzman SJ (2008) Dropsy, dialysis, transplant: a short history of failing kidneys, Johns Hopkins biographies of disease. University Press, Baltimore

Pliny the Elder, Healey J (1991) Natural history: a selection. Book XXVI: disease and their remedies. Clay Limited, St. Ives, p 244

Reed JA (1954) Aretaeus, the Cappadocian. Diabetes 3:1

Sagesaka H, Sato Y, Someya Y et al (2018) Type 2 diabetes: when does it start? J Soc Endocrinol 18(20 5):476–484

Schaaf HS (2009) Renal tuberculosis. In: Tuberculosis: a completes clinical reference. W.B. Saunders, Elsevier, Philadelphia

Schneider D, Lilienfeld DE (2008) Public health: the development of a discipline: from the age of Hippocrates to the progressive era. Rutgers University Press, New Brunswick

Sheela CG, Augusti D (1992) Antidiabetic effects of S-allyl cysteine sulphoxide isolated from garlic. Indian J Exp Biol 30:523–526

Strassler RB, Purvis AL (2008) The landmark Herodotus: the histories. Anchor Books, Random House Publishing Group, New York

van Dieren S, Beulens JWJ, Grobbee DR (2010) The global burden of diabetes and its complications: an emerging pandemic. J Cardiovasc Prev Rehabil Suppl 1:S3–S8

von Straden H (2007) Herophilus: the art of medicine in early Alexandria: edition, translation and essays. Cambridge University Press, New York

Wootton D (2006) Bad medicine: doctors doing harm since Hippocrates. Oxford University Press, New York

Zhu KY, Guo SS, Liang XC (1983) Diabetes mellitus treated by traditional Chinese medicine. J Am Coll Tradit Chin Med 1:24–30

Zucconi LM (2007) Medicine and religion in ancient Egypt. Relig Compass 1(1):26–37

2

A Disease of the Kidneys

The weakening of the Western Roman Empire generally marks the beginning of the Early Middle Ages, with a decline in historical records and advancements. Known as 'The Dark Ages' from the fifth to tenth centuries A.D., this period saw a return to bartering as a form of generalised currency when money became scarce with the departure of the Roman legions. Those who could left with the legions for protection, heading to the Roman frontier (Kaufmann and Kaufmann 2001). During this time, physicians returned to their home countries, taking with them their medical experience and skills (Wilkinson 2001).

The departure of doctors, coupled with societal disruption, brought medicine to a standstill. In the Western European world, this would last for more than 500 years (Castleden 1994). While the Church and monasteries preserved some ancient medical texts, progress in understanding and treating illness declined, and access to healthcare was limited, with many relying on traditional healers or religious figures. However, the Eastern world, and Islamic and Byzantine civilisations continued to advance knowledge of diabetes, although the kidneys were still felt to be the main cause.

What was formerly the Western Roman Empire had now fallen into the 'Dark Ages', and although there was some use of common medical practices, much had regressed to the use of folklore. The use of magic had little effect on diseases that swept across Europe, not having much else to rely on as a 'cure' for ill health (Dawson 2005). Despite this, Greek physicians *Oribasius*, *Alexander of Tralles* and *Paul of Aegina* continued their use of traditional methods and understanding at this time (French 2003).

V. Wilson, *Diabetes Ancient and Modern*, Hippocrates,
https://doi.org/10.1007/978-3-032-12454-8_2

The late Middle Ages (thirteenth to fifteenth centuries A.D.) saw a decline in feudalism, the Black Death and The Hundred Years' War. Despite this, the expansion of European thinking during the Crusades signalled advancement in areas such as teaching and studying at monastic centres, aiding population growth and commerce.

The Orient

Medical thinking and learning in China during this period advanced only by rational ideas rather than by examination of the inner human body, as it was forbidden on religious grounds under the system of beliefs and practices supported by Confucius and his fellow philosophers, leading to a reduction in medical and biological progress (Dan 2010). The purpose of human organs still centred around the existence of the four bodily humours, with the belief that each emotion was based in a certain organ of the body, creating a new fifth humour (Yanchi 1995).

General Medical Treatments

During the Dark Ages in China, treatment of disease involved a blend of traditional practices, and early forms of public health measures. Emphasis continued to be placed on balancing yin and yang and using herbal remedies, with the use of early forms of quarantine, isolation and public health initiatives to combat epidemics. Other remedies included massage and dry-cupping, which made blood readily available for bloodletting. Acupuncture was used to relieve pain and congestion, and cautery to scorch the skin, where a preparation of burning oil-soaked Chinese wormwood leaves was applied to boils and lesions, and to address infections (Hong-Yen and Peacher 1978).

Rhubarb was regarded as an effective laxative, while aconite (a drug from a poisonous plant, especially monkshood), arsenic and opium were combined with animal extracts with an established significance in ancient customs (Bensky et al. 2004). To treat diabetes, ginseng was relied upon to reduce sweetness in the body. This practice is based on some truth, while other remedies listed in the Chinese *Materia Medica*—a comprehensive body of knowledge documenting the substances used in traditional Chinese medicine—have now been shown as having no useful benefit and were rejected (Bensky et al. 2004). Aside from ginseng, a further 22 other herbs were mentioned in Chinese medical texts to reduce sweetness in the body (Yanchi 1995).

A fasting remedy was also employed to treat the symptoms of diabetes, this being the oldest treatment for most causes of disease adhered to in every religion (Lloyd and Sivin 2004). This would have helped people with type 2 diabetes to lose weight, potentially reversing the symptoms, but this was not a long-term sustainable option.

Today, valuable contributions from Chinese medicine provide beneficial treatments. Used conventionally for patients with thyroid swelling, seaweed—containing iodine—had a valuable effect on reducing the growth; willow bark was a source of pain-relieving salicylic acid—the active component of modern-day aspirin, and rutin was sourced from mulberry flowers, used as an effective treatment for high blood pressure (Bensky et al. 2004).

Chinese society has always emphasised the need to care for the poor and destitute, especially during illness. An increase in Buddhist practices during the Hang Dynasty (206 B.C.–220 A.D.) and the T'ang Dynasty (618–907 A.D.) saw the advancement of hospitals where patients could stay and be treated by Buddhist physicians. Early healthcare in the Buddhist tradition was provided in monasteries, particularly in Sri Lanka, where they were established as early as the fourth century B.C.

These hospitals offered a blend of medical and spiritual healing, and some even featured advanced medical practices like surgery and acupuncture. Anti-Buddhist sentiment would, in the ninth century, take control, forcing the closure of more than 4600 hospitals and temples of healing. This halted any further progress in providing healthcare for the general public for more than 300 years (Lloyd and Sivin 2004).

Physicians

According to Yanchi (1995), there were four types of Chinese physician:

- The chief physician, who made up prescriptions for drug remedies, and tested the skills of other physicians.
- Physicians who treated minor ailments, such as headaches, colds and small wounds.
- Physicians with surgical skills who treated larger wounds and bone fractures.
- Those who studied animal anatomy and treatments.

A physician would have treated patients with diabetes symptoms, advising on six types of food and drink to restore health (Lloyd and Sivin 2004). Physicians would mainly treat patients with type 2 diabetes thought to have been caused by a poor diet with an excess of greasy foods. It was standard practice for Chinese doctors to make reports regarding all patient outcomes, both good and bad. These reports helped maintain the high standards of medical practice and reduce the number of unqualified practitioners, as all reports had to be submitted to the authorities (Yanchi 1995). By the seventh century A.D. physicians needed to have passed examinations in order to practice (Lloyd and Sivin 2004).

Dissemination of knowledge was a common practice within Europe. However, in China, acquired medical knowledge was only passed to others who studied this discipline, and their immediate family who wished to follow in their footsteps (Hong-Yen and Peacher 1978). A physician would teach his student free of charge, not being concerned with financial gain as he passed on his knowledge. Tuition fees were later introduced by the courts; the master was directly responsible for the actions of his pupil, paying a fine if the student did not pass their medical exams (Hong-Yen and Peacher 1978).

Diagnosis

Eastern physicians employed diagnostic methods which included taking the patient's pulse, and while conversing, noting the patient's speech patterns and physical mannerisms. These practices were widely used in many civilisations to gain as much information about the patient as possible to indicate the cause of disease or ill health.

In China, the root of all disease was felt to be not showing appropriate reverence to the Tao—'the principle of staying happy and calm under all circumstances' (Hong-Yen and Peacher 1978). The Tao encompasses mind, body and spirit and follows a holistic approach regarding the patient's welfare not only in their standing in life, but also in all aspects, including their diet, dreams, employment, family and friends.

The earliest written records mentioning taking the pulse as a diagnostic method appear in the Nei Jing, also known as the Huangdi Neijing, which is attributed to the Yellow Emperor and is thought to date back to around 698–589 B.C. This text emphasises the importance of pulse examination in assessing a patient's health and disease state. It was standard practice to measure the patient's pulse in both wrists, comparing it to that of the doctor for normality. This diagnostic technique had the advantage that the patient could remain fully clothed. It was also thought important for the doctor to note the time, date and season as it was believed that the pulse rate changed hourly (Lloyd and Sivin 2004).

Each pulse beat was divided into three stages, these having both a shallow and a deep prominence attributed to various organs within the body (Lloyd and Sivin 2004). In ancient Greece, Galen suggested a similar theory in his book, *The Pulse for Beginners*, which described the pulse as having three qualities of length, breadth and depth (Wootton 2006). The Pulse Classis or *Mai Jing* was written by *Wang Shuhe* in the 3rd century A.D. (Yanchi 1995).

Human Anatomy

As we have seen in the ying-yang principle of Chinese medicine, the kidneys were believed to be two parts of the whole. The left kidney produced urine, while the right was 'the gate of life' containing the jing—spirit essence. This belief was expanded to describe reproduction: the right kidney in males stored the 'essence', while the right kidney in females contained the womb. Early Chinese medical texts speak of the kidneys in the context of the testes (Yanchi 1995). It was later understood that each bodily organ plays an individual role. With this in mind, *Sun Szu-miao* (581–682 A.D.) wrote the foremost medical text Qianjin Yaofang (*Chin Yao Fang*) translates to something very close to A *Thousand Golden Remedies* or more formally *Essential Prescriptions Worth a Thousand Pieces of Gold*, a 30-volume medical treatise containing the sum of recognised medical knowledge (Lloyd and Sivin 2004).

Symptoms

Zhen Li-yan (589–618 A.D.) wrote his important medical text during the Sui Dynasty. *Efficacious Formulae Recorded from Antiquity to the Present* recognised the main symptoms of diabetes as 'frequent thirst that leads to excessive drinking, excessive urination, and urine that is sweet and without fat' (Lloyd and Sivin 2004). This work was based on Zhen Li-yan's observations regarding the consistency of diabetic urine.

By the year 752 A.D. it had been established that diabetic urine contained sugar (glucose) as stated by *Wang Tao* in his book, *Wai tai mi yao / Wang Tao* (*A Collection of Diseases*). However, diabetes is only one of 1100 other diseases included in the text (Lloyd and Sivin 2004).

If a patient was suspected of having diabetes, Wang Tao suggested that they test their urine daily by urinating 'onto a wide, flat brick to observe whether any ants gathered to collect the sugar'. In an advanced way, he recommended that a record was kept of ant activity. Physicians throughout Asia recommended urination onto a pile of sand to observe whether this attracted insects, naming diabetes the 'sugar-urine disease' (Lloyd and Sivin 2004).

Wang Tao also recommended that people with diabetes eat pork pancreas, an early and incredibly forward-thinking recognition that the pancreas is involved in the onset of diabetes. Wang Tao managed diabetes in his patients using observation. Urine that did not contain excessive amounts of sugar saw no insect activity.

Glucose is excreted in the urine when the blood glucose level reaches 10 mmol/L (or 180 mg/dL in the USA).

Beliefs About Diabetes

Chinese medicine held that excess heat in the body was the cause of disease. In this respect, physician *Liu Wansu* (1120–1200 A.D.) suggested that diabetes should be treated with herbal remedies of a 'cold nature' (Yanchi 1995). Traditional Chinese Medicine has a similar approach today, where diabetes can be treated with herbal remedies to disperse heat and nourish the yin (Bensky et al. 2004). Liu Wansu documented herbal remedies to reduce sweetness with formulae designed to help with obesity and type 2 diabetes (Yanchi 1995).

Diseases that were very rare, like type 1 diabetes, might never be encountered in a physician's career. Some conditions were not recorded, such as type 2 diabetes with symptoms that were often ignored. Some types of illness were attributed to a different cause, especially diabetes being classed as a disease of the kidneys. Later, health problems were named according to their symptoms, with diabetes being known as the 'sugar-urine disease' (Dawson 2005).

Between the sixth and eighth centuries A.D. medical knowledge continued to spread throughout Asia (Durant 1950). Japanese scholars travelled to China to study medicine; by the late eighth century a medical school had been founded, and Chinese medicine became firmly established in Japan (Lloyd and Sivin 2004). Further medical teachings based on Islamic Arabic texts were translated from Sanskrit into Chinese, and vice versa, helping the distribution of medical knowledge throughout India and the Arab-speaking world (Durant 1950).

The Persian Empire

With the expansion of the Islamic Empire in the seventh century, many medical texts became available to them. These were translated into Arabic from Greek, Indian, Chinese and Syrian (Durant 1950). This spurred the developing Persian Empire into a flourishing centre of learning, concentrated within the central cities. Medicine was just one area in which scientific advancements were made.

With the decline and final destruction of the library in Alexandria, texts that had been readily available were no more. It is fortunate that many Arabic scholars had previously translated these texts (Nutton 2005). Scholars and physicians now followed the newly converted Greek and Roman medical texts, and were known as Arabists (Ardalan et al. 2008), bringing new interest in the area of diet and health.

With the growth of the Islamic Empire in the twelfth century came a renewed interest in progressing the field of medicine within Europe (Nutton 2005). One particular text, commonly known as *The Learner's Guide to Medicine*, included diseases of the kidneys and urinary tract, providing much-needed knowledge, although diabetes was still seen as such a disease (Medvei 1993).

Treatment

Islamic principles maintained 'that God did not send down a disease without also sending down a cure', which included diabetes. The physician, *Isaac Judaeus* (932 A.D.) wrote the first book containing only dietary guidance (Miller et al. 2010a). In the twelfth century, *Maimonides* wrote several popular works on diet and hygiene (Maimonides 2004). *Al-Quareshi* (1213–1288), also known as Ibn al-Nafis, wrote essays on diet and eye diseases, such as cataracts (Miller et al. 2010b). It is due to these Arabist scholars that advancements were made in all areas of medicine, especially ophthalmology (eye care) and nutrition.

The preservation of health was a widespread concern, and the health-giving benefits of a proper daily routine regarding correct diet, exercise and rest became very popular. Medieval physicians took a full life history from the patient to determine the suspected cause of the illness, as well as measuring the pulse and examining the urine (Nutton 2005). Herbal remedies were common, especially for treating symptoms of diabetes, with a total of 92 types of medical herbs prescribed to treat diseases of the urinary system and bladder

(Ardalan et al. 2008). These remedies targeted excessive urination, rather than the cause—too much glucose in the blood, spilling over into the urine.

Galen's medical knowledge was still seen as important, even in the twelfth century. Renowned Jewish physician, philosopher and rabbi, Maimonides (1135–1204) revived 1500 pieces of earlier written advice to achieve a healthy lifestyle (Wootton 2006). Maimonides documented having seen more than 20 cases of diabetes, claiming them to be due to 'sweet waters of the Nile and excess heat that spreads across the kidneys' (Maimonides 2004).

His works on diet and hygiene extend to 21 'common sense, enduring rules'. Rule two advises the avoidance of excess food to 'overload the stomach', and that when eating a meal, the patient should be 'content with less than necessary to make him feel quite satisfied' (Maimonides 2004). This practical advice is as relevant today as it was then.

Those suffering from a loss of health were advised to follow the special rules for their particular disease or condition, only to be found in his own medical books. In Rule 20, the physician also observes that 'every change in life habit is the beginning of an ailment' (Maimonides 2004), which is true of type 2 diabetes in cases triggered by poor diet and infrequent exercise.

The great Persian physician, Abu Bakr Muhammad Bin Zakaria Razi, known to the West as *Rhazes* (865–925), wrote 232 medical essays combining knowledge from ancient texts with his own experience, creating *Liber Continens* (*The Continent* or *The Comprehensive Book on Medicine*). In the *Kitab al-Hawi*, Rhazes translates the known Indian information about diabetes, providing complicated treatments for this condition, frequent urination and obesity. Like Maimonides, Rhazes also stated that dietary management was key to the treatment of obesity, suggesting that diabetes was 'a warm, functional disease of the sex organs' (Medvei 1993).

Kitab al-Hawi was translated into Latin and reprinted numerous times, becoming highly influential across Europe (Nutton 2005). This comprehensive medical encyclopaedia was completed by followers of Rhazes after his death. This extensive work had analysed the medical thinking of all major civilisations on every aspect of the progression of disease.

Eighth to Ninth Centuries

The practice of herbalism became widespread during the eighth century A.D., freeing up physicians who had traditionally dispensed these remedies (Dawson 2005). Physicians were now able to concentrate solely on diagnosing disease, and follow-up visits to see if the health of a patient was improving with a particular treatment. Pharmacology—defined as the scientific study of drugs and how they affect living organisms—then became a specialised science and profession in its own right, gathering understanding of the 'chemical properties of remedies prescribed for all diseases', including diabetes (French 2003).

Kitab-al-Malik was a prominent work by *Haly Abbas* (died 994 A.D.), addressing both the theory and practice of medicine to become a standard medical text (Georgacarakos 2011). Christian translators introduced the work of Haly Abbas to the West, his writings on anatomy becoming the basis of medical knowledge for the next 300 years (Durant 1950). Similar to Maimonides and Rhazes, Haly Abbas thought diabetes arose from an excess of heat in the body (viscus), calling the condition 'dysentery of the discrepancy' (Ardalan et al. 2008).

Tenth to Twelfth Centuries

The development of hospitals is due to the contribution of Islamic medicine to the Western medical tradition, where the prefix 'hosp' denotes a place providing care, hence the words 'hospice', 'hospital' and 'hospitality' (Dawson 2005). As we have seen, hospitals originated from Buddhist monastic infirmaries in the sixth to ninth centuries, but instead of providing care for the general public, these places cared for monks in poor health, or for those who had undergone purification by being bled.

Several centuries later, monasteries paid doctors to visit them (French 2003). Every monastery had accommodation for travellers and pilgrims, and some priories eventually developed into dedicated hospital facilities, providing healthcare to travellers and townsfolk. As with the spread of ideas through Muslim advancement, so grew the use of monastic guesthouses, which were attributed to the Crusades (1099–1291), with the provision of charity as part of the Christian ethos (Nutton 2005).

The tenth-century Islamic 'Father of Surgery', Al-Zahrawi (*Albucasis*), wrote a description on the couching operation to remove the lens of an eye clouded with cataract (Georgacarakos 2011). *On Surgery and Instruments* states: 'the surgeon should take the couching instrument in his left hand to treat the right eye, and vice versa, plunging the blade in at the edge of the patient's cornea covering the front of the eye, using a rotating motion to achieve penetration of the white tissue' (Lewis and Spink 1973).

This surgery was performed without the use of anaesthesia; anaesthetic was not introduced until the nineteenth century. The writings of Albucasis show a detailed understanding of the anatomy of the eye, correctly identifying that a clouded lens behind the pupil would cause poor vision. Sushruta in ancient India, and Celsus (25 B.C.–50 A.D.) had documented this procedure much earlier.

Avicenna (980–1037 A.D.) was a Persian doctor, philosopher and scientist. Although only 40 of his medical texts still survive, Avicenna is believed to have produced 450 works on the subjects of medicine and philosophy. Similar to Rhazes in the fourth century, *Qhannon fel teb of Avicenna* (The *Canon of Medicine*), completed in 1025, gathers together all aspects of medical understanding (Avicenna 2005).

The Canon of Medicine is a summary of Persian, Chinese and Indian medical practice, attempting to place Galen's medical theories within Aristotle's natural philosophy—the principle of form and matter, the four causes, the rigid separation of the world into opposed spheres and the finite nature of the universe. This accessible textbook was so popular, scholars no longer consulted the original sources of medical thinking:

- Book one of the Canon contains detailed descriptions of anatomy and physiology, showing how the body works.
- Book two discusses diseases and ailments of the body 'from top to toe'.
- Book three focusses on treatment and cure. Avicenna also listed 760 uncompounded medicaments in his *De Materia Medica* (Wootton 2006).

What of Diabetes?

With the availability of food and the associated increase in obesity, Avicenna documented the rise in type 2 diabetes. In *The Cannon of Medicine*, Avicenna describes diabetes and its causes, including the rarer diabetes insipidus. He encouraged the tasting of patients' urine, naming this 'aldulab', or water wheel, noting the excessively sweet taste of the urine in uncontrolled diabetes: 'when the urine of diabetics is left to stand in ambient air, it leaves a residue that is particularly sticky and tastes sweet as honey' (Avicenna 1997).

Avicenna describes in detail his theory on the cause and treatment of low blood glucose levels—known medically as *hypoglycaemia*, and if severe, hypoglycaemic coma. When patients had high blood glucose levels—known medically as *hyperglycaemia*—he prescribed concoctions to make his patients vomit. References to 'primary' and 'secondary' types of the disease distinguish between type 1 and type 2 diabetes, and several chronic complications were recognised in association with high glucose levels in untreated diabetes, including blindness and loss of sexual function.

Herbal remedies, exercise and a specific diet were prescribed by Avicenna as a treatment for diabetes, in conjunction with emetics to make the patient sick, and sudorific drugs to cause sweating. As diabetes was believed to be a disease of the kidneys, Avicenna prescribed these drugs to alter fluid levels in the body. Although this is Galenic medicine and humoural balance, Islamic physicians believed that disease could be treated in more than one way, incorporating beliefs from other cultures (Georgacarakos 2011).

As a form of exercise, Avicenna advised diabetic patients to ride on horseback to 'employ moderate friction' (Avicenna 1997). Any repetitive exertion was thought to bring health benefits. The lifespan of someone with type 1 diabetes without insulin was just over 12 months. For those with type 2 diabetes, who survived longer, Avicenna wrote in *The Canon of Medicine* that patients should take 'tepid baths and fragrant wine'. Herbs listed as useful in reducing the sweetness of urine included lupin, Trigonella plant (fenugreek) and zedonary seeds (Medvei 1993). Various spices were frequently used in Arabic remedies, such as nutmeg, cloves and mace.

The advancement of hospitals to provide care saw both medical and surgical wards, a pharmacy, clinics, a library, lecture theatre, chapel and mosque, although the emphasis was on medicine rather than religion. By 1225, *Abd al-Laṭīf al-Baghdādī* (1162–1231) had written the first essay dedicated solely to diabetes (Ardalan et al. 2008).

The Thirteenth Century

Persia was invaded by the Mongols in the thirteenth century, ceasing advances in medicine as many libraries and medical texts were destroyed. Persian medicine continued with few notable advances until it was outdated by Western medicine in the nineteenth century (Nutton 2005). *Avenzoar* (1090–1162) questioned historical medical thinking concerning the dominance of Galen's humoural theory (Elliot 2008).

The Mongol destruction of Bagdad in 1258 A.D. (Castleden 1994) signified the end of medical advancement in Persia. The study of anatomy declined along with doctors and hospitals. Consequently, medical knowledge did not advance further for another 600 years, when it was surpassed by European medical thinking in the nineteenth century.

Doctors became known as physicians in the thirteenth century if they had completed a university education (Wootton 2006). The basic theories on human anatomy and disease did not change until the role of bacteria and viruses in the spread of disease was gained in the early nineteenth century

(Wootton 2006). Several medical terms introduced by the Arabs have remained in Western languages, such as 'syrup', 'drug', 'alcohol' and 'alkali', and many new aspects of herbal medicine were introduced and improved (Nutton 2005).

The Byzantine Empire

Medicine in the Byzantine world is a vast, under-researched topic. The history of Byzantine medicine falls into two periods of enlightenment. Alexandrian medicine governed the first period, with its unrivalled medical and philosophical scholarship heralding substantial discoveries in the Greek-Byzantine world (Miller et al. 2010a). This was brought to an end in 642 A.D. with the Arab conquest of Alexandria. The second period from 642 to 1453 marked the expansion of medical understanding and practice, where distinguished physicians conducted research (Eftychiadis 1997). The teachings of Hippocrates and Galen still had some influence in this new era.

Diagnosis in the Fourth to Fifth Centuries

From the late fourth century A.D. the inspection of urine (*uroscopy*) became common practice in Byzantium (now known as Istanbul, Turkey). Instead of making a diagnosis by physically examining the patient, uroscopy became the alternative, so the physician didn't even need to be in the same room as the patient when assessing their illness, proving popular in the diagnosis and prognosis (outcome) of almost every health condition (Diamandopoulos 1997). Only a surgeon would touch the patient when operating (Wootton 2006).

Byzantine physicians built upon the teachings of Galen in order to offer comprehensive explanations for kidney and bladder disorders; diabetes still being regarded in this way. The second Byzantine period concentrated on the search for truth, rather than magic and curses being a cause of disease, consequently uroscopy gained popularity as a diagnostic tool (Eftychiadis 1997).

More advanced thinking pulled away from ancient Greek beliefs, and followed the idea that a sensible diet and exercise were the route to good health. Using scientific methods to examine the urine enabled the detection of diabetes, as well as other diseases. Aretaeus of Cappodocia documented the dilute appearance and frequency of urination in diabetes. To assist with observing the appearance of urine in a glass flask, several tests were developed for this purpose (Diamandopoulos 1997), including those to:

- Examine glassy sediments.
- Detect opacity.
- Observe concentration, colour and smell.
- Look for any pus residues.

Between the fourth and seventh centuries A.D., prominent physicians wrote on the subject of uroscopy: Oribasius, Aëtius of Amida, Stephanus of Athens and *Paul Eginetus*. The study of uroscopy continued to be valued into the thirteenth century, where Theophilus Protospatharius wrote the famous *Peri ouron* (Angeletti and Cavarra 1997).

Minute changes in the kidney cells that preceded any symptoms of diabetes was first discovered by *Oribasius* (325–beginning of the fifth century A.D.), such as hardening of the kidney tissue in *nephropathy*—diabetic kidney disease (Eftychiadis 1997). The Greek physician performed anatomical dissections, forming the belief that the role of the kidneys was to attract urine from the blood, theorising that diabetes was a type of dropsy, with excess fluid gathering within tissues and cells.

Without the confines of strict rules on dissection, Oribasius was able to describe the circulation of the blood, although this is chiefly attributed to William Harvey in 1628. Spanish physician *Michael Servetus* wrote *The Christianismi Restitutio* (*Restoration of Christianity*) in 1553, the year of his death (Lovci 2008). This contains what is believed to be the first description of the minor (pulmonary) circulation: the part of the circulatory system that carries deoxygenated blood from the heart to the lungs, returning oxygenated blood back to the heart.

Oribasius described diabetes insipidus as a rare disorder of the pituitary gland, observing that an afflicted patient could drink as much as 10 litres of water a day (Miller et al. 2010a). *Liber Passionalis* is devoted entirely to diabetes mellitus and insipidus (Grant 1997), where Oribasius recognises that type 1 diabetes is a disease occurring most often in childhood, in contrast to type 2 diabetes onset in adulthood (although type 2 now also occurs in children due to a poor diet and inactive lifestyle).

Treatments in the Fourth to Fifth Centuries

Oribasius documents that 'obesity is a pathological condition requiring treatment which brings about emaciation in the patient through fat reduction'. Similar to Chinese beliefs, he prescribed a treatment for obesity (and type 2 diabetes) that altered the patient's 'temperament to warm rather than moist', which would 'render the individual lean'. Regular exercise, herbal medications, baths, massage and 'provocation of mental anxiety' was also recommended for weight loss (Grant 1997). Previous thinking held that an excess of heat (anger and frustration) was the cause of diabetes, meaning that Oribasius thought differently in advising that a 'warm temperament' (friendly and approachable behaviour) would reverse the symptoms of diabetes.

Significant advances in the treatment of ill health took place, with the use of 'tablets placed under the tongue, saline solutions, nasal powders, and calming gases' (French 2003). Plant and animal extracts were used to treat disease, such as, 'camphor, musk extracts from animal glands, arsenic, mercury, and borax' (Georgacarakos 2011). Usage of traditional medical herbs continued for the treatment of diabetes, with humoural theory still explaining the cause of the disease. Drugs were only believed to work effectively in combination with a healthy lifestyle, supplemented with purging and cleansing remedies (Nutton 2005).

Byzantine physicians believed obesity to be a problem of the endocrine glands (Medvei 1993), prescribing 'diet, purging, bloodletting, physiotherapy, bathing, and diuretics such as parsley and cinnamon to reduce the appetite' (Khan et al. 2003). Recognising that type 2 diabetes is often obesity-related is forward-thinking.

Sixth Century

Stephanus of Athens wrote two books on uroscopy, analysing the colour of urine according to humoural theory. He was also interested in where and when the urine was passed as a diagnostic tool (Angeletti and Cavarra 1997). In terms of diabetes, Stephanus considered that the patient's urine could provide information about past, present and future ill health (Nutton 2005).

Stephanus considered blood was present in the body for lubrication, its dense consistency also sustaining the heart, lungs and other organs before being 'attracted to the kidneys from the large vein [vena cava] and becoming urine by passing into the bladder' (Angeletti and Cavarra 1997).

Stephanus also observed, 'like blood, like urine' (Eftychiadis 1997), referring to the overspill of glucose into the urine in diabetes. We know from ancient texts that untreated or miss-managed diabetes results in higher levels of sweetness. Stephanus stated: 'perfect function affords pure urine and imperfect function results in urine of poor composition', when referring to the function of the liver, although this also applies to regulating blood glucose levels. However, Stephanus could not have known that one function of the liver is to convert and store excess glucose.

Aetius of Amidas devoted one section of his medical encyclopaedia, *Tetrabiblon*, to diseases of the kidneys, diabetes, bladder stones and venereal disease (Miller et al. 2010a). Aetius recommended that the patient be bled and given diuretics at the onset of diabetes, both treatments intended to purge 'excess' water from the body. Aetius described two urinary conditions: 'dysuria, when the patient has desire and passes urine with difficulty'; and 'strangury, where urine is passed in drops' (Diamandopoulos 1997).

Writing several books, including one describing the value of uroscopy in diagnosing the severity of disease, Aetius compared the urine of a healthy individual with that of the patient, analysing these samples according to humoural theory (Diamandopoulos 1997). Patients with type 1 diabetes—generally felt to be a 'fat-melting disease with too much heat should produce black, oily urine in conjunction with an excess of black bile' (Duffy 1984).

The texts that followed reported which properties of urine best explained the disease, although this led to some physicians describing false and inaccurate colours of urine which did not aid correct diagnosis. The number of colours of urine described towards the end of the Byzantine era had reached twenty (Diamandopoulos 1997).

Treatments in the Sixth Century

Aetius recommended the use of garlic in the treatment of diabetes, for its blood glucose-lowering effects, also examining the appearance of the patient's blood for qualities such as 'fatness' (Miller et al. 2010a)—perhaps describing high sugar content. The loins on a human are the sides of the body between the lower ribs and the hips (Medvei 1993). This continues the belief that excess heat in the body can bring about diabetes.

For those in the later stages of type 1 diabetes, drowsy, with muscle wasting and dehydration affecting organs and tissues, and immense pain, Aetius used opiates such as poppy juice and mandragora (Georgacarakos 2011), a narcotic plant with large yellow fruit from the mandrake family. High blood glucose over time causes damage to the nervous system (diabetic *neuropathy*), a painful and chronic condition.

Sixth-century Greek physician and independent scientist, *Alexander of Tralles*, wrote *The Practice of Medicine* and several other medical texts. As a skilled practising pharmacist, he prescribed iron for the treatment of anaemia, and rhubarb for liver weakness (Elliot 2008), showing his acute understanding of effective remedies.

Alexander suggested that diabetes was greatly helped with a diet that was difficult to digest, including foods such as 'the feet of oxon, the flesh of pompions [an old word for pumpkins], and chestnuts' (Medvei 1993). This way of thinking was possibly an attempt to use some of the excess glucose during the digestive process; Alexander did not agree with the use of diuretics to remove excess fluid from the patient, and he did not mention cutting the veins (*venesection*) to remove disease.

Similar to Aretaeus (250 B.C.), Alexander of Tralles prescribed oil of roses (oleum attar) and myrtle to cure 'defluxation' (Elliot 2008). Defluxation is defined as 'an excessive or abnormal flow from any of the natural openings' (Whittles and Whittles 1994). This describes perfectly the symptoms of excessive urination in diabetes, considered a 'difficult medical problem' by Alexander of Tralles, especially in childhood. Oil of roses has no therapeutic value in diabetes, but a moderate diet and regular exercise is recommended for people with the condition.

Ninth Century

Paulus Aegineta (Paul of Aegina) wrote extensively on diabetes, stating that (Paulus Aegineta 1844):

> Diabetes is the rapid passage of the drink out of the body, liquids being voided by urine as they were drunk and hence it is attended with immoderate thirst; and therefore, the affliction has been called dipsacus, being occasioned by weakness of the retentive faculty of the kidneys while the attractive is increased in strength and deprives the whole body of its moisture and immoderate heat.

We can see that raised body temperature is again believed to be the cause of diabetes symptoms, as previously documented in other accounts. A lack of insulin can indirectly contribute to overheating or make it harder to regulate body temperature. Insulin plays a role in regulating body heat and glucose uptake, potentially leading to overheating or making it more difficult to cool down.

In his herbal and plant remedy with no carbohydrate (which breaks down into glucose for fuel) and a little protein, Paul of Aegina recommended that the patient take a mixture of 'pot-herbs, endive, lettuce, rock fishes, juices of knotgrass, elecampane [a plant with bitter leaves and root] in dark-coloured wine and decoctions of dates and myrtle' for newly diagnosed diabetes (Paulus Aegineta 1844). He also warns against using diuretics as patients were already losing too much fluid, although he did advocate bloodletting. In the later stages of the disease, he prescribed 'cataplasms [poultices] to the area of the abdomen below the ribs over the kidney consisting of vinegar, rose oil and navelwort'.

Paulus concentrated much of his work on diseases of the kidneys and described a treatment for frequent urination consisting of 'bread, birds, sea urchins, vegetables, eggs, fennel, celery, and carrots' (Miller et al. 2010a). When compared with his treatment for the onset of diabetes, this prescribed a low-fat diet with balanced proteins and vegetables. This diet would have been a permanent lifestyle change to treat and reverse obesity and associated type 2 diabetes.

Thirteenth to Fourteenth Centuries

Humoural theory underwent another modification in the thirteenth century A.D., adding the signs of the zodiac to the concept of the four humours, using the patient's date and time of birth to aid the diagnosis of disease (Elliot 2008). In Ancient Greece around 300 B.C., zodiac signs were attributed to a particular part of the body, where Aries ruled the head, Gemini ruled the shoulders and so on. The zodiac constellations also influence the onset of certain illnesses—Pisces, Cancer and Capricorn caused diseases with sores, scales and fistulas (abnormal tunnels between body parts and skin), while Sagittarius and Gemini were responsible for falling fits and seizures.

Folk medicine used birthstones to protect against disease, and if a patient was scheduled for surgery, their month of birth was avoided as it was believed this would not bode well for both the treatment and subsequent healing (Heindel 2010). Even as late as 1332, the horoscope was consulted before bleeding patients (Wootton 2006). Those being trained in medicine studied astrology as a significant factor of health and wellbeing, medicine and astrology being seen as one and the same. The ambiguities of astrology protected the doctor, as negative astrological projections could be blamed if a treatment did not work.

As mentioned earlier, *Theophilus Protospatharius* was the author of the famous *Peri ouron*, the leading text on the examination of urine (Angeletti and Cavarra 1997). The inspection of urine was now being used as a means to diagnose disease, whereas previously it was only used to assess disease outcome. He was also one of the first to examine narrowing of the blood vessels at the level of the tissues.

Theophilus Protospatharius categorised urine in the following ways (Wallis 2000):

- Whether the liquid appeared thick or thin.
- Its colour in the range of white to black (pale, dilute urine indicating diabetes).
- The presence of any sediments and their position in the urine.

Joannes Actuarius produced *De Urinis* (On Urines) and *De medicamentorum compositione* (On the Composition of Medicaments), a seven-book discourse on the qualities of urine. Although he was also a physician, Actuarius is Latin for a notary, record-keeper or clerk. Seeming to ignore the work of his contemporaries, Actuarius stated that he had written his seven books because 'the subject had never been fully investigated by ancient authors' (Miller et al. 2010a). His work provides analysis of the different states of urine, diagnosis, reasons for this occurrence and prognosis of urinary disease (Diamandopoulos 1997).

He also explained four types of digestion—one phase giving a description of diabetes which is similar to that of Aretaeus (250 B.C.), detailing how 'flesh and limbs are melted down into urine' and the transformation of 'blood to flesh' (Duffy 1984).

Advancing the practice of uroscopy, Joannes Actuarius invented a uroscopy vial 'made of good quality translucent glass'. This ruled out any imperfection in the glass, allowing good observation and any abnormalities in the urine. Actuarius also advocated that additional information, such as the measurement of the pulse, should be included to make a comprehensive diagnosis (Miller et al. 2010a).

The study of uroscopy was so professionally important that documentation needed to be carried to prove ability to practice; this standardisation first occurred in Syria. In Jerusalem in 1245, according to law, a doctor 'should be whipped around the streets' if a patient died (Wootton 2006). Similarly, if ever a 'urine doctor' was discredited, he was required to carry his urine flask through the streets (Diamandopoulos 1997).

Europe

Before the Muslim influence in Europe, Europeans followed archaic beliefs in relation to the cause of disease. They relied on prayer and visiting shrines containing holy relics for the relief of their symptoms. Later Christian monks founded hospitals (Sirass 1990). In the twelfth century two key hospitals were built in England for the recuperation from illness: St Thomas' in 1100 and St Bartholomew's in 1123 (Hollingham 2008).

Thirteenth Century

Human dissection was allowed for medical examination and to determine cause of death, and strict public hygiene measures were brought in to control the spread of disease (Dawson 2005). Religious establishments had a great belief in fasting remedies to cure 'an excess of waste and poisons in the body', which they saw as a result of dietary excess and little exercise (Crawford and Lee 2010). It was thought that resting the organs of elimination, (the kidneys, bowels and skin) by fasting allowed the body to heal itself.

Palma and Bologna universities developed into leading centres of medical teaching and learning in the thirteenth century (Crawford and Lee 2010). After the dissolution of the monasteries in the sixteenth century, these establishments eventually evolved into famous medical schools. Schools of medicine were also founded in Salerno, Italy; Montpellier in southern France; and Bologna in Padua (Crawford and Lee 2010).

Fasting remedies for diabetes—still being regarded as a disease of the kidneys at the time—were probably effective for those with type 2 diabetes.

> Today, risk factors such as obesity and taking little or no exercise are often cited as reasons for the escalating epidemic of people worldwide developing type 2 diabetes (Wilkinson 2022).

Fourteenth Century

In 1315 a climatic change in the form of a mini ice age swept across Europe. This resulted in a dramatic reduction in available food, lasting for more than 2 years as widespread flooding followed (MacDougall 2006). The famine brought about a decline in obesity and associated type 2 diabetes and heart disease (Crawford and Lee 2010).

As the population of the world increased, epidemics swept freely across the continents. Half a million people died in 1319 during a typhoid epidemic (Bartlett 2010), followed by The Black Death—seen as a judgement by God—which swept across Europe and reached England by 1348, when three million people died (half the population), including physicians (Ormrod and Lindley 1996).

There was little progress in medical understanding, and with other pressing issues, little time to devote to the investigation of diabetes. Public health measures saw vast improvements in an effort to curtail the spread of disease. Philosopher Roger Bacon (1214–1292) stated that 'medicine should rely solely on chemical remedies in order for it to become a scientific and consistent discipline' (French 2003).

Summary

There was no notable progress in the understanding and treatment of diabetes during the Early and Late Middle Ages. Despite this, several diagnostic and more scientific blood and urine tests allowed diabetes to be recognised earlier and managed as well as possible with herbal and plant medicine.

In the Eastern world, Persia and Byzantium, diabetes was still regarded and treated as a disease of the kidneys and bladder due to frequent urination. The overarching belief of imbalance in the four bodily humours as a reason for disease meant that diabetes was often treated with bleeding or purging. By the twelfth century, those with ill health, including diabetes, could be treated in the first hospitals, upgrading medicine from the use of herbal remedies in the home to a scientific practice, dedicated to treating the causes of disease and the management of chronic long-term conditions.

References

Angeletti LR, Cavarra B (1997) The *Peri ouron* treatise of Stephanus of Athens: Byzantine uroscopy of the 6th–7th centuries A.D. Am J Nephrol 17:228–232

Ardalan MR, Shoja MM, Tubbs S et al (2008) Diseases of the kidney in medieval Persia – the Hidayat of Al-Akawayni. Nephrol Dial Transplant 10:1093

Avicenna (1997) The Cannon of medicine (book three, part 3), Translated into Persian by A. Sharafkandi (Hajar). Soroush Press, Tehran

Avicenna (2005) The metaphysics of the healing (Islamic translation series): a parallel English-Arabic text translated, introduced and annotated by M.E. Marmura. Brigham Young University Press, Utah

Bartlett E (2010) The history, diagnosis, and treatment of typhoid and typhus fever: with an essay on the diagnosis of bilious remittance and yellow fever. Nabu Publishing, Bibliobazaar/BiblioFile, South Carolina

Bensky D, Clavev S, Stodger ER (eds) (2004) Chinese herbal medicine: Materia Medica, 3rd edn. Eastland Press, Seattle

Castleden R (1994) World history: a chronological history of dates. Parragon Book Service Limited, London

Crawford S, Lee C (2010) Bodies of knowledge: cultural interpretations of illness and medicine in medieval Europe: studies in early medicine Volume 1, British Archaeological Reports International Series. Archaeopress, British Archaeological Reports, Oxford

Dan Y (2010) Confucius from the heart: ancient wisdom for today's world. Pan Books, London

Dawson I (2005) Medicine in the middle ages. Hodder Wayland, China

Diamandopoulos AA (1997) Uroscopy in Byzantium. Am J Nephrol 17:222–227

Duffy J (1984) Byzantine medicine in the Vth and VIth centuries: aspects of teaching and practice. Dumbarton Oaks Papers

Durant W (1950) Age of faith (the story of civilization). In: The story of civilization Part IV. The Book Service, Colchester, pp 162–186

Eftychiadis AC (1997) Diseases in the Byzantine world with special emphasis on nephropathies. Am J Nephrol 17:217–221

Elliot JS (2008) Outlines of Greek and Roman medicine. Bibliobazaar/BiblioFile, Charleston

French, R. (2003) Medicine before science: the business of medicine from the middle ages to the enlightenment. Cambridge: Cambridge University Press

Georgacarakos M (2011) Ancient traditional medicine of Byzantine, Egypt, Greece, Medieval, Islam, Iran, and Rome. Lightening Source UK, Milton Keynes

Grant MD (1997) Dieting for an emperor: translation of books 1 and 4 of Oribasius' medical compilations with an introduction and commentary. E.J. Brill, Boston

Heindel M (2010) The message of the stars: an esoteric exposition of medical and natal astrology, exploring the arts of prediction and diagnosis, 3rd edn. L.N. Fowler and Company, London

Hollingham R (2008) Blood and guts: a history of surgery. BBC Books, Ebury Publishing, Random House Group, London

Hong-Yen H, Peacher WG (1978) Chen's history of Chinese medical science. Oriental Healing Arts Institute, Long Beach

Kaufmann JE, Kaufmann HW (2001) The medieval fortress: castles, forts and walled cities of the middle ages. Greenhill Books, London

Khan A, Safdar M, Nuzzafar M et al (2003) Cinnamon improves glucose and lipids of people with type 2 diabetes. Diabetes Care 25:3215–3218

Lewis MS, Spink GL (1973) El Zahrawi on surgery and instruments, English translation and commentary. The Wellcome Institute of the History of Medicine
Lloyd G, Sivin N (2004) The way and the word: science and medicine in early China and Greece. Yale University Press, London
Lovci R (2008) Michal Servetus, heretic or saint? CreateSpace, Seattle
MacDougall D (2006) Frozen earth: the once and future story of ice ages. University of California Press, London
Maimonides M (2004) Medical aphorisms: treatises 1–5, Complete medical works of Moses Maimonides. University of Chicago Press, London
Medvei VX (1993) The history of clinical endocrinology. The Parthenon Publishing Group Incorporated, New York
Miller FP, Vandrome A, McBrewster J (eds) (2010a) Byzantine medicine: Byzantine empire, Islamic medicine, medical compendium in seven books, Paul of Aegina, Vienna Dioscurides, Oribasius, Nicholas Myrepsos. Alphascript Publishing, Beau Basin
Miller FP, Vandrome A, McBrewster J (eds) (2010b) The Cannon of medicine: Avicenna, Avicennism, the book of healing, Unani, Ibn al-Nafis, Abu al-Qasim al Zahrawi, Al-Tasrif, medical literature, Avicenna (crater), Ibn Sina Peak, Pharmacopeia. Alphascript Publishing, Beau Basin
Nutton V (2005) Ancient medicine (science of antiquity series). Routledge, Taylor and Francis Group, London
Ormrod M, Lindley P (1996) The Black Death in England, 1348–1500. Paul Watkins Publishing, Lincolnshire
Paulus Aegineta (1844) The seven books. F. Adams, London
Sirass, N.G. (1990) Medieval and early renaissance medicine: an introduction to knowledge and practice. London: University of Chicago Press
Wallis F (2000) Inventing diagnosis: Theophilus' *De Urinis* in the classroom. DYNAMIS Medical Scientific History Illustrated 20:31–73
Whittles KH, Whittles CA (1994) Claremont medical dictionary. Claremont Books, London
Wilkinson P (2001) What the romans did for us. Bath Press Limited, Bath
Wilkinson E (2022) World health assembly ratifies first global diabetes targets. Lancet Diabetes Endocrinol 10(8):560
Wootton D (2006) Bad medicine: doctors doing harm since Hippocrates. Oxford University Press, New York
Yanchi L (1995) The essential book of traditional Chinese medicine: volume 1: theory. Columbia University Press, New York

3

The Renaissance

With the development of the printing press by Thomas Caxton (1422–1491) combined with the high-quality wood-cut illustration of Johannes Gutenberg (1400–1468), medical textbooks were quickly copied and circulated, helping to promote standard medical practices. The printed word would eventually be promoted via a network of libraries, where any educated person could view these texts.

Those that could not read still believed that magic and witchcraft were the source of disease. In the sixteenth and seventeenth centuries, a physician might provide an acceptable opinion, instead of a medical treatment. In Italy, experimentation combined with observation brought about scientific conclusions. This re-established the need to find a cause and treatment for the major diseases that periodically swept across Europe. As such, diabetes was not the priority, but in 1425, the term 'diabete' was first seen in the English language.

Fourteenth to Fifteenth Centuries

With the development of scientific knowledge came the need to revise all previous medical thinking. As a result, Galen's dominant theories once again re-emerged and were translated, being irrefutably absorbed into 'modern' European medical thinking (Johnston 2006). The Renaissance brought about a new interest in human anatomy, although this was mainly through artistic interpretation, rather than through medicine (Rifkin et al. 2011).

V. Wilson, *Diabetes Ancient and Modern*, Hippocrates,
https://doi.org/10.1007/978-3-032-12454-8_3

The Resurgence of Humoural Theory

The four humours theory of blood, yellow bile, black bile and phlegm had been prominent for 2000 years. With the revival of Galen's beliefs, physicians once again blamed disease, including diabetes, on imbalance in the body (Wootton 2006). Students of medicine were expected to read Galen's works and follow them without question (Johnston 2006). Although this had no basis in healing, humoural theory outweighed all other ideas on health and illness. Those suffering from diabetes were 'continually bled and prescribed emetics to make them vomit' (Medvei 1993). These treatments merely served to weaken the individual and hasten their death.

Dissection

Post-mortem dissection to establish cause of death had occurred prior to 1300 (Richardson 1988). Religion has always played a part in the dissection of the human body, sometimes in favour of the practice, and other times against it. In 1315, *Mondino de Luzzi* taught anatomy by public dissection of criminals. However, this practice was not common.

The term 'dissection' was known as anatomy in the sixteenth century (Wootton 2006). The first public dissections became standardised under *Vesalius* in the mid-sixteenth century, and by the eighteenth century, every medical student was expected to have performed human dissection. This led to a shortage of available bodies, and the practice of body-snatching. Practical anatomy allowed physicians to discover where the organs are positioned in the body. It is this development that finally brought about the dispelling of humoural theories as these new anatomists could readily see the diseased organs and tissues before them (Hollingham 2008).

Leonardo da Vinci (1452–1519) was one of the greatest creators of human anatomical drawings. He was enthralled by all the structures within the body, and would make liquid wax casts as accurate representations of these structures (Rifkin et al. 2011). Much of Leonardo's work was lost and remained unpublished during his lifetime, but eventually contributed greatly to the understanding of the human body (Wootton 2006).

Understanding Drugs

Knowledge of the types and uses of drugs increased rapidly during the Renaissance era, and opiates, such as laudanum, and anaesthesia were commonly used to control pain (Snow 2008). Since the time of the ancient Greeks, herbalists had used a variety of ingredients to make their potions and pills. However, it was not known which of these ingredients were actually effective.

Due to the rise in population and the ease by which contagious diseases could spread, it became a priority to pinpoint the substances with beneficial effects to combat this problem. Girolamo Fracastoro published his seminal work on contagion, *De contagione et contagiosis morbis et eorum curatione* (On Contagion and Contagious Diseases, and Their Cure), in 1546. Knowledge and practice of more advanced surgical procedures also progressed and was made possible with the use of anaesthetics (Wootton 2006). Humoural thinking had been superseded by modern anatomical knowledge, incorporating the long-held belief in observation and scientific methods to study disease.

Sixteenth Century

Religious teachings held that disease was caused by evil and demonic possession (Holland 1590). In their search for answers, lay persons turned to university-educated doctors for insight (Thomas 1971). In sixteenth-century Europe, physicians finally accepted that diabetes caused the loss of more fluid than the patient could take in, heralding a new desire to discover the reason for this loss.

Paracelsus (1493–1541) was a Swiss alchemist and doctor. He had already dismissed humoural theory, focusing instead on chemical methods to provide insight into the origins of disease (Patcher 2008). He substituted chemicals for the four elements, concluding that some diseases lay outside the body, although not diabetes (Paracelsus and Waite 2009). By recognising that each disease required a different treatment, Paracelsus was unique.

Paracelsus disagreed with the study of urine as a diagnostic tool, going as far as to burn classical medicine texts and shunning ancient Greek theories (Ball 2007). He described diabetes as 'a constitutional disease that irritates the kidneys and provokes excessive urination' (Eknoyan and Naqv 2005). Although this regards diabetes as a disease of the kidneys, it suggests an alternative reason for great thirst and urination associated with the condition.

Paracelsus tasted diabetic urine to detect the presence of sugar, recording that evaporation of the urine resulted in an 'excessive residue of abnormal white powder'. Wrongly documenting this residue as 'salts' rather than sugar, he believed this to be the cause of the patient's thirst. He later wrote (Paracelsus and Waite 2009):

> Diabetes is an affliction of the blood being involved with salt particles [where these particles] do not run through the most open passages of the Reins [kidneys].

> This is a close description of how the body deals with an excess of glucose by passing it out with the urine, although the residue in urine was not identified as glucose until the seventeenth century (Medvei 1993).

Similar to Paracelsus, *Andreas Vesalius* (1514–1564) challenged Galen's ideas. This maverick anatomist cut down a body from the gallows with the intention of boiling it down to bare bones; he later reassembled the skeleton using wire so he could study it, continuing this practice over many years (Hollingham 2008). He became Professor of Anatomy at the University of Padua in Italy. The act of removing a body hanging from the gallows to use for dissection was illegal, but little was ever said about where the bodies of criminals stolen for anatomical research ended up (Richardson 1988).

In 1543, Vesalius published *De humani corporis fabrica libri septem (On the Fabric of the Human Body in Seven Books)* (Wootton 2006). With the use of dissection, Vesalius gained a thorough understanding of human anatomy. He also wrote, *De Humani Corporis Fabrica* (*The Fabric of the Human Body*), a seven-volume medical work in 1543; this work was illustrated using the best artists from Titian's studios (Wootton 2006).

Vesalius described the pancreas (although he did not call it this) as having 'a protective function for the stomach as it lays across the abdomen' (Vesalius 1988). In 1541, Vesalius sketched the human pancreas, including the main duct (Vesalius and Albinus 2008). This was first described in detail by *Johann Georg Wirsung* in 1642 after the dissection of a rooster's pancreas (Howard and Hess 2002).

Proving Galen wrong on over 300 areas of human anatomy that had previously been based on animals, Vesalius argued that students should only draw conclusions from human anatomical studies. Despite this, the renaissance in anatomical thinking spread slowly through Europe, with Galen's hold still evident well into the nineteenth century, even though printed medical texts were widely available (Wear 1981).

The first book published in the English language was *The Method of Physicke* by Elizabethan surgeon, *Dr Philip Barrough* in 1583; this later went into seven editions (Pelling and Webster 1979). His work was a summary of all medical knowledge, including diabetes, although at the time 'demonic poisons' were felt to be a major factor in all diseases which needed to be purged. This included bloodletting and the use of senna pods and warm beer (Butterfield 1950). Barrough's book contained no new insight on the treatment of diabetes.

Seventeenth to Eighteenth Centuries

The innovation of the microscope (1670s–1680s) allowed us to view a previously invisible world, although the term 'microscope' was first applied to describe one of *Galileo's* instruments in 1625. In 1661, *Marcello Malpighi* (1628–1694), known as the founder of microscopic anatomy, used this method to study the 'minute biological structures of the lungs' (Wootton 2006). *Giovanni Alfonso Borelli* (1608–1679) was an Italian physiologist who researched the microscopic constituents of the blood and glands (Stawart 2011). However, microscopic information was not seen as a valuable contribution to science; it was not until the 1830s that the relevance of the unseen world was revered (Wootton 2006).

Borelli and Malpighi founded an Italian scientific academy in 1657. Malpighi advanced our understanding of the causes of diabetes with his microscopic studies of the glands (Meli 2011), being the first to observe and report minute structural changes in the body (a science known as histology), and to examine the capillaries and their relationship with the arteries and veins (Butterfield 1950). Malpighi also provided detailed descriptions of complex internal structures, such as the pancreas, overturning the idea that the organs were 'shapeless lumps formed out of congealed blood' (Wootton 2006).

Due to premature mortality, some people may not have lived long enough to develop type 2 diabetes, as average life expectancy in the seventeenth century was mid-thirties (Siraisi 1990). There were specialists in the treatment of diabetes, but few could afford them, while the Church perpetuated the belief that 'illness was good for the soul'.

Nicholas Culpepper (died 1697) learnt his apothecary trade in the plague-ridden streets of London. With his knowledge of Latin, Culpepper translated the *Pharmacopoeia* (an official publication listing medicinal drugs, their effects and directions for use) into English. Although he had not completed his herbalist training, he practised illegally in Spitalfields, calling himself a 'physician for the ordinary man'. Here, he tried to cure the ills of up to 40 patients every morning (Wooley 2004).

Culpepper brewed tea from the herbs tansy and willow to treat diabetes. He also used white willow to prevent vomiting, which was useful in the treatment of patients with type 1 diabetes (Culpepper 1981). Willow herb (epilobium angustifolium-L) was also used as a laxative, driving out impurities from the body. Scorning the use of uroscopy, Culpepper believed that it was better to physically examine a patient than to observe their urine from a distance, stating: 'to look upon the body is far better than to look on as much piss as the Thames might hold' (Culpepper 1981).

Culpepper believed that astrology strongly influenced health and disease, where the organs of the body were ruled by the position of the planets. Naming the astrological characteristics of medicine 'decumbiture', this influence on health and disease distinguished Culpepper as a unique thinker among apothecaries (Wooley 2004). This belief put Culpepper at odds with current thinking. With the discovery of germs under the microscope, the germ theory of disease was established in 1865. This gave little opportunity for doctors to use astrological alignments as a reason for illness and treatment failures.

Following the death of Charles I in January 1649, censorship of medical publications was lifted and without this restriction, Culpepper's earlier translation of *Pharmacopeia* became widely available. He then produced *The English Physician's Guide to Herbal Medicine*, telling his publisher that the book must be priced at 3 pence per copy to make it affordable to everybody (Culpepper 1981). His book sold so well that it remained in print for 300 years.

Pathology

Following in the footsteps of Vesalius, *Giovanni Battista Morgagni* (1682–1771) also became Professor of Surgery and Anatomy at Padua University, Italy. Described as the Father of Pathology, he believed that disease was a result of an alteration in the organs. *De Sedibus et Causis Morborum per Anatomen Indagatis* (On the Seats and Causes of Diseases Investigated by Anatomy) is the seminal 1761 masterpiece by Giovanni Battista Morgagni (Morgagni 1986). Having carried out over 400 dissections, Morgagni observed that each organ should be regarded as a 'composite of minute mechanisms'.

Documenting his thoughts on diabetes, he observed that: 'What is drunk should be discharged by the urinary passages without the least changes whatsoever, preserving the same colour, consistence, taste and smell as when taken in'. At the time Morgagni was writing, red wine was the favoured drink to quench the thirst due to poor water quality; the resulting urine would still have been pale and dilute due to the quantity of fluid consumed. Morgagni believed that the symptoms of diabetes were due to 'internal damage to the digestive organs'. He promised that he would find the harm that diabetes had caused to the body at post-mortem (Morgagni 1986).

Treatments

Doctors often claimed that the medicine or treatment they had prescribed was responsible for the patient's recovery, when much of this was actually due to natural healing. In 1657, less than one tenth of patients were cured by a doctor (Wootton 2006). The placebo effect—a drug that has no medical benefit, but is believed to work by the patient—can improve the health of one third of those who take them, especially if the doctor is confident of the treatment's effect (Wootton 2006).

Advancing the Understanding of Diabetes

The Renaissance period saw the progress of medical research, especially the investigation of human anatomy at cell level under the microscope. Doctors and physicians were willing to try any method to reduce the symptoms and suffering of their patients with diabetes. There were two opinions on how best to treat diabetes in the seventeenth century (Wheeler 2000). One treatment involved replacing the sugar that was lost in the urine; the other involved dietary restrictions of what we now know to be carbohydrates, recognised as a class of compounds in 1844. Dietary remedies for the treatment of diabetes at that time were often high in carbohydrates, and low in calories. This was the case until the nineteenth century, when both high and low carbohydrate diets were equally recommended for the treatment of diabetes (Wheeler 2000).

Sylvius a famous Dutch physician and scientist examined the role of bile and pancreatic juice in digestion, believing the pancreatic duct secreted directly into the intestine (Chen and Chen 1995). *Regnier de Graaf*, who studied under Sylvius, analysed pancreatic juice extracted from the pancreatic duct in dogs. Sylvius observed that the secretion tasted bland and acidic. De Graaf did the same experiment with human pancreatic juice, declaring that it had the same taste as canine pancreatic secretions.

Johann Conrad Brunner (1653–1727) also studied the pancreas, observing that after a dog's pancreas was removed, the animal could live for up to one year, although it showed symptoms of frequent urination, excessive thirst and vomiting (Medvei 1993). If only Brunner had tested the dog's urine for sugar, a link between diabetes and the pancreas could have been made much sooner.

Having discovered the circle of cerebral (brain) blood vessels named after him, the English brain physician, Professor *Thomas Willis* (1621–1675), working at Guy's hospital in London, wrote his diabetes classic *The Pissing Evil.* Willis regarded diabetes in this way because his patients would pass an average of 10–15 quarts (almost nine and a half to fourteen litres) of urine each day (Furdell 2005).

For a long time, physicians believed that diabetes was a disease related to the blood, kidneys, liver or stomach, failing to recognise that the true cause of diabetes is insulin deficit. Stating that diabetes was rare in centuries past, Willis made a number of perceptive observations about type 2 diabetes, including that it occurred with over-consumption associated with a rich diet (Willis 1678):

> In our age, given to good fellowship and gusling [guzzling] down chiefly of unalloyed [rich] wine, we meet with examples and instances enough, I may say daily, of this disease … wherefore the urine of the sick is so wonderfully sweet, or hath an honeyed taste… As to what belongs the cure, it seems a most hard thing in this disease to draw propositions for curing, for that its cause lies so deeply hid, and hath its origin so deep and remote.

Willis' experiments confirmed previous knowledge that sugar from sweet foods was passed into the urine. He also concluded that these sugary excretions were not present in healthy individuals, but only in those suffering with diabetes. With the import of sugar increasing rapidly by the mid- to late seventeenth century, type 2 diabetes was no longer a rare condition in the richer classes. At the time Willis was King Charles the Second's physician. This placed him in a difficult position with the growing number of wealthy people developing type 2 diabetes due to the import of sugar that the king made a huge revenue from.

Willis recommended dietary restrictions for patients with type 2 diabetes, suggesting that his wealthier patients ate only barley, bread, milk and water, although this was not welcomed and rarely adhered to (Hughes 2009).

Thomas Willis was so sure that diabetes began within the blood and not the kidneys, he wrote (Willis 1678):

> It in no way pleases us that some do assign for the cause of Diabetes the attracting force of the Reins [kidneys]: because the Blood is not drawn to the Reins but driven thither by the motion of the Heart. Further neither doth Serum seem to be drawn or emulged from Blood washing through them, but to be separated (as we have already more clearly shewed) partly by straining, and partly by fusion or a certain kind of precipitation: wherefore we believe the Diabetes to be rather and more immediately an affection of the Blood than the Reins.

We now know that stress can increase blood glucose levels because the liver releases glucose in preparation for confrontation. Thomas Willis was the first physician to recognise this effect, proving it was possible to create an increase in blood glucose by subjecting patients to 'emotional or physical upset'. This experiment showed that glucose levels increase for reasons other than eating (Willis 1678).

Thomas Sydenham (1621–1675) believed diabetes must occur on the minute level (meaning at cellular level) in the body (Wootton 2006). Similar to Willis, Sydenham was sure that diabetes originated in the blood, and was undoubtedly due to poor digestion and absorption. The product of this irregular digestive process was 'chyle' that resulted in diabetes as it could not be emitted from the body (Sydenham 1978). Together with scientist John Locke, Sydenham wrote *Observations on Fevers and Acute Diseases* (Sydenham and Locke 1669).

Pieter Pauw, a Dutch anatomy professor, concluded from his records of diabetes cases that there was a difference between what we now know as type 1 and type 2 diabetes according to body shape (Singer 1957).

Scientists and physicians in the seventeenth century continued to make advances towards an understanding of diabetes as a disease, and how the patient's body is affected. Advances in understanding diabetes pointed tantalisingly towards the involvement of the pancreas, and a substance that somehow controlled blood sugar (glucose) levels.

Summary

The Renaissance in medical understanding finally moved beyond humoural theory as the definitive cause of all diseases. Without a reliable chemical test, tasting the urine and blood of patients with diabetes to detect a 'honeyed taste' was the only way to monitor excess glucose. This remained the case until the beginning of the twentieth century. Whilst there was still no effective treatment for the symptoms of type 1 or type 2 diabetes, both conditions continued to be eased with a modified diet and herbal remedies.

Scientific methods using objective experiments rather than relying on subjective opinions were used to explore the cause of diabetes. Renaissance doctors renewed their interest in discovering how and why this condition developed. Andreas Vesalius' publication of *De Humani Corporis Fabrica Libri Septem* saw the beginning of a new era in medicine, involving a break with the old traditions and ways of thinking. This paved the way for the modern scientific experimental age in which the cause of diabetes could finally be identified.

References

Ball P (2007) The devil's doctor: Paracelsus and the world of renaissance magic and science. Arrow Books, Random House Publishing Group, London

Butterfield H (1950) The origins of modern science. Bell and Sons Limited, London

Chen TS, Chen PS (1995) The history of gastroenterology: essays on its development and accomplishments. The Parthenon Publishing Group, New York

Culpepper N (1981) Culpepper's complete herbal and English physician, Facsimile reprint edition. Harry Sales

Eknoyan G Naqv J (2005) A history of diabetes mellitus, or how a disease of the kidneys evolved into a kidney disease. Science Direct. https://www.sciencedirect.com/science/article/abs/pii/S1548559505000261

Furdell EL (ed) (2005) Willis and Sydenham on diabetes: discovery and debate in early modern English medicine. In Textual healing: essays on medieval and early modern medicine. Studies in medieval and early reformation traditions (110). E.J. Brill, Boston

Holland H (1590) A treatise against witchcraft, Cambridge University Press

Hollingham R (2008) Blood and guts: a history of surgery. BBC Books, Ebury Publishing, Random House Group, London

Howard JM, Hess W (2002) A history of the pancreas: mysteries of a hidden organ. Springer, New York

Hughes JT (2009) Thomas Willis: 1621–1675: his life and works. Royal Society of Medicine Press Limited, London

Johnston I (2006) Galen: on diseases and symptoms. Cambridge University Press, London
Medvei VX (1993) The history of clinical endocrinology. The Parthenon Publishing Group Incorporated, New York
Meli, D.B. (2011) Mechanism, experiment, disease: Marcello Malpighi and seventeenth-century anatomy. Baltimore: Johns Hopkins University Press
Morgagni GB (1986) Sedibus et Causis Morburnum per Anatomen Indogatis, Acta Encyclopedica 6. Encyclopedia Italiana
Paracelsus, Waite AE (2009) The hermetic and alchemical writings of Paracelsus – two volumes in one. Martino Press, Connecticut
Patcher H (2008) Paracelsus – magic into science. Hesperides Press, London
Pelling M, Webster C (1979) Medical practitioners. In: Health, medicine and mortality in the sixteenth century. Cambridge University Press, Cambridge
Richardson R (1988) Death, dissection and the destitute. Phoenix Press, London
Rifkin BA, Ackerman MJ, Falkenberg J (2011) Human anatomy: depicting the body from the renaissance to today. Thames and Hudson, London
Singer C (1957) A short history of anatomy and physiology from the Greeks to Harvey. Dover Publications, Mineola/New York
Siraisi N (1990) Medieval and renaissance medicine: introduction to knowledge and practice. University of Chicago Press, Chicago
Snow SJ (2008) Blessed days of anaesthesia: how anaesthetics changed the world. Oxford University Press, New York
Stawart DTC (2011) Giovanni Alfonso Borelli: Renaissance, Physiology, Physicist, Mathematician, Galileo Galilei. Betascript Publishing, Beau Basin
Sydenham T (1978) The works of Thomas Sydenham. Gryphon Books, New York
Sydenham T, Locke J (1669) Observations on fevers and acute diseases. Papers held by the Royal College of Surgeons
Thomas K (1971) Religion and the decline of magic: studies in popular beliefs in sixteenth and seventeenth century England. Weidenfeld and Nicholson, London
Vesalius A (1988) De Humani Corporis Fabrica, Bilingual edition, Latin America. Octavio
Vesalius A, Albinus L (2008) Classic anatomical illustrations. Dover Publications, New York
Wear A (1981) Knowledge and practice in English medicine, 1550–1680. Cambridge University Press, Cambridge
Wheeler ML (2000) Cycles: Diabetes nutrition recommendations—past, present and future. Diabetes Spectr 13(3):116–121
Willis T (1678) Pharmaceutice Rationalis or an exercitation of the operations of medicines in human bodies. Dring, Harper and Leigh, London
Wooley B (2004) The herbalist: Nicholas Culpepper and the fight for medical freedom. Harper Collins, London
Wootton D (2006) Bad medicine: doctors doing harm since Hippocrates. Oxford University Press, New York

4

Is it Glucose?

With the rejection of Galen's humoural theory, combined with scientific advancements, such as the microscope, progress in medicine and anatomy moved at a pace. Greater emphasis was now being placed on the causes of disease. New chemical tests were beginning to develop, and surgery was becoming safer due to the advancement of anaesthetics. Despite this significant progression, the cause of disease was still often attributed to magic, or 'miasma theory', where poisonous vapours in the air were thought to seep from rotting matter, causing disease. This theory was based on the observation that disease outbreaks often occurred in areas with poor sanitation and foul odours.

The pressing medical concerns of the day dictated research into diseases such as smallpox, meaning finding the cause of diabetes was less urgent. Although becoming more prevalent, some doctors were still uncertain about using new scientific techniques, preferring to stick to what they knew. This unwillingness to change perceptions slowed the advance of diabetes research, leaving many questions unanswered.

Detecting Glucose

Physicians had for many centuries realised that patients with diabetes produced sweet urine. However, it was not until 1774 that chemist *Robert Wyatt* proved beyond doubt that blood and urine samples contained a type of sugar, rather than salts or acids. This understanding was further advanced in 1815

V. Wilson, *Diabetes Ancient and Modern*, Hippocrates,
https://doi.org/10.1007/978-3-032-12454-8_4

by *Eugene Chevreuil*, who correctly identified the sugar present as glucose (Brock 1992).

One of the first studies of a patient with diabetes mellitus in the scientific age is attributed to Matthew Dobson (1735–1784). His subject, Peter Dickinson—a 33-year-old soldier, was considered to have 'typical' diabetes symptoms. In 1772, Dickinson was admitted to the Liverpool Infirmary hospital for observation, and was noted as 'suffering from extreme thirst, excessive urination, weight loss, and dry skin', indicating he had advanced type 1 diabetes.

It is documented that Dickinson was passing 28 pints of urine per day which is three-and-a-half gallons of fluid, or almost 16 litres. Thomas Willis had previously documented a similar finding, observing that his patients would pass an average of 10–15 quarts (almost nine and a half to fourteen litres) of urine each day. After this research was seen by contemporaries belonging to a medical society, Dobson's findings were promptly published to circulate this remarkable observation in the medical society journal (Dobson 1776).

His research paper was based on nine patients with diabetes. Five experiments were carried out using the blood and urine of Peter Dickinson, from which Dobson concluded eight research findings. Although this may have been 'tested' by taste alone, rather than by any chemical means, the second experiment explains his method and conclusions (Dobson 1776):

> Eight ounces of blood taken from the arm of this patient exhibited, after standing a proper time, the following appearances… The serum was opaque, and much resembled common cheese whey; it was sweetish, but I thought not so sweet as the urine.

Later, he wrote:

> Two quarts of this urine were, by gentle heat, evaporated to dryness, under the inspection of Mr. Poole, apothecary to the hospital, and Mr. Walthall, one of the house apprentices. There remained after evaporation, a white cake which was granulated, and broke easily between the fingers; it smelled like brown sugar, neither could it, by the taste, be distinguished from sugar, except that the sweetness left a slight sense of coolness on the palate.

In the conclusion of his five experiments, Dobson states that Peter Dickinson's urine had 'very little of the nature or sensible qualities of urine', as it was so dilute. Dobson summed up in his fifth experiment that 'a considerable quantity of saccharine matter is removed by the kidneys in every case of diabetes' (Marwood 1973). Similar to Thomas Willis' findings, the glucose in Dickinson's urine was seen to have originated from his blood, rather than his kidneys.

Advances in Understanding

Referring to a patient with type 1 diabetes, Dobson wrote: 'I have known it terminate fatally in less than five weeks'. He also observed that the disease had a longer path in some patients, in reference to cases of type 2 diabetes (Dobson 1776).

Dobson correctly recognised that the reason patients with type 1 diabetes were so thin was because their bodies were unable to use the food they had consumed, causing rapid weight loss. Food taken in was 'drawn off before it could be applied to the purposes of nutrition'. As such, 'the only sensible cure is to strengthen the patient's digestive powers, to promote a due sanguification [formation of blood cells in the living body], and to establish a perfect assimilation throughout the whole economy' (Dobson 1776).

Dobson recognised that future research was important to determine how carbohydrates were broken down into glucose. As such, he believed that biochemistry should become an independent science (Morgan 2004).

Dobson's Treatments

Peter Dickinson was required to regularly eat quantities of rhubarb and senna pods as a purging remedy to 'keep the body constantly open'. Dobson also recommended that Dickinson took the healing waters of Matlock in Derbyshire, offering to pay for this treatment. Dickinson, now in an advanced weakened condition through purging methods and untreated diabetes, refused any further treatment, including Dobson's rhubarb cure.

Dobson dismissed Dickinson's lack of improvement as the fault of his severely ill patient, suggesting he must have 'mis-applied the treatment given for his relief', and therefore probably 'felt ashamed that he had not followed his doctor's advice properly' (Dobson 1776). Dobson's inability to 'cure' Dickinson was also explained by the obvious worsening of the condition as Dickinson's diabetes entered a final stage towards the end of his life.

Types of Diabetes

Following on from the advancements of Wyatt and Dobson, *John Rollo* (1758–1809) was a Scottish doctor and Surgeon General in the Royal Artillery. Considered to be an expert, John Rollo concurred with Dobson that diabetes was unquestionably a disorder arising from 'a stomach dysfunction'. Both Rollo and Dobson agreed sugar was being lost in the urine because it couldn't be used for nutrition (Morgan 2004). Rollo developed a successful 'dietary treatment' where patients were fed 'an animal diet of blood pudding and meat that is fat and stale' (Wheeler 2003). In this way, Rollo's patients were eating protein and fat on this diet, but no carbohydrates.

> Although not known at the time, consumed carbohydrates break down to eventually form glucose, an excess of which then passes from the blood into the urine via the kidneys.

Rollo stated that diabetes was specific to the absorption of 'saccharine matter in the stomach' (Withers and Wood 2002). He examined the effectiveness of different types of diet for people with diabetes in England, and thereafter the condition was widely known as 'diabetes anglicus', despite the fact that much of Rollo's clinical research took place in France and Germany.

Recognising Complications

From ancient times it became apparent that diabetes also brought with it other serious health problems.

> We now know that these health issues are triggered by high blood glucose levels in body cells. Even for people with diabetes today who take insulin and have good diabetes self-management, the duration of diabetes means that body cells are affected over time by this altered metabolism, and complications are triggered.

Frederick William Pavy (1829–1911) was a nineteenth-century London physician. He wanted to advance the treatment of diabetes by understanding its nature, basing this work on his many patients with type 2 diabetes. The advancement of hospital care meant that by 1789, most patients were no longer seen in their own homes (Wootton 2006). Pavy's research extended over a number of years to observe the progression of diabetes, the onset of any complications and how long these patients survived.

Pavy's research showed that the presence of glucose in both the blood and urine was automatic: if it appeared in the blood, it would also be seen in the urine (Pavy 1862). Pavy was able to observe that many of his chronically ill patients had consistently raised glucose levels, and was able to clearly establish a causal link between diabetes and its secondary complications, especially nerve damage in the extremities.

Pavy dedicated so much time to finding the cause of diabetes that Queen Victoria's physician, William Gull, commented: 'What sin has Pavy committed, or his fathers before him, that he should be condemned to spend his life seeking a cure for an incurable disease?' (Pavy 2009). As there was still no cure for diabetes, the only option for nerve pain was to prescribe opium treatment, which continued until 1915 (Bliss 1988).

Dietary Treatments

Though advancements in understanding diabetes had been made, in the late 1850s, *Pierre Adolphe Piorry*, a French physician, continued to believe that lost sugar should be replaced (Morgan 2004). Piorry had found that his patients with diabetes were rapidly losing glucose and believed that the answer lay in restoring this balance.

It is not known whether Piorry questioned the cause of excessive glucose excretion. The sugar replacement diet caused the death of several patients, and Piorry was discredited and no longer allowed to practice medicine. Another physician supporting the replacement of lost sugar then became diabetic himself. He followed his own advice, consumed large quantities of sugar and died shortly afterwards (Bliss 1988).

As had already been noted, eating carbohydrates increased the sweetness of the patient's urine. *Ludwig Traube* (1818–1876) a German physician, confirmed this idea (Miller 2010). He also went on to confirm that the use of a restricted diet, where carbohydrates were limited, resulted in less glucose being excreted; although he did not specify how this was measured, this was most probably achieved by simple chemical analysis. Traube also realised the importance of body temperature in disease, and as a diagnostic tool, introduced thermometers to Berlin hospitals in 1850 (Wootton 2006).

During the Franco-Prussian War at the siege of Paris in 1870 when food was scarce, the French physician *Apollonaire Bouchardat* observed that patients with type 2 diabetes often had little or no glucose in their urine. Seeing this as a potential dietary cure, despite disagreement from some of his patients, he introduced periodic fasting days. Bouchardat realised that regular exercise helped to substantially reduce glucose levels, allowing modest intake of carbohydrates without a sharp increase in blood glucose, stating 'you shall earn your bread by the sweat of your brow' (Bliss 1988). Bouchardat concluded that an increase in glucose levels was in direct proportion to carbohydrates consumed, and that a considerable reduction in carbohydrates, coupled with regular exercise was a viable treatment for type 2 diabetes. He also helped to plan individual eating regimes to maximise his patients' health (Morgan 2004).

There were several other notable physicians who recommended dietary remedies for diabetes. *Catoni*, an Italian diabetes specialist, went so far as to lock the rooms of his patients, thus enforcing his dietary restrictions upon them. Catoni noted that his regime 'prevents the patient from falling into a diabetic coma and adds a few more months to his or her life' (Morgan 2004). This harsh treatment was also imposed by German physician, *Bernard Naunyn* (1839–1925) who imprisoned his patients for 5 months so they could obtain 'sugar freedom' (Bliss 1988).

An oat-based diet was introduced by fellow German physician, *von Noorden* in 1902 as an approach to treating diabetes by reducing glucose. Recognising that oats are digested slowly and do not cause a sharp rise in blood glucose, this diet was similar to modern day, allowing patients to eat more oat-based carbohydrates (Bliss 1988).

The 'starvation diet' of 500 calories a day became the most effective way to reduce glucose levels (Allen 1915). There was still the persisting belief that what was lost needed to be replaced. *Frederick Madison Allen* (1879–1957), a leading American diabetes consultant, stated that it was necessary to sweep away 'the modern fallacy of replacing through the diet the calories lost in urine' (Bliss 1988).

Allen believed that previous treatments had been ineffective because they attempted to substitute fats for carbohydrates, leading to diabetic ketoacidosis, coma and death. He found that a liquids-only diet could avoid high glucose levels and acidosis in diabetes patients. In the early stages of a diabetes diagnosis, eating a low-carbohydrate diet would have been of benefit to patients, but it would not have saved their lives.

It was believed that achieving a reduction in glucose meant the patient was cured. However, if they ate 'normally' again, their blood glucose levels increased once more. Many doctors saw wealthy patients with type 2 diabetes as a good source of income, so it was advantageous to keep them alive with restrictive diets for as long as possible—potentially reversing their condition with weight loss. Patients with incurable type 1 diabetes, however, gained little or nothing from these dietary restraints.

The Body's Use of Glucose

The metabolism of glucose occurs in 10 successive chemical reactions, including what is medically known as glycolysis, the most crucial process in releasing energy from glucose for the body to use as fuel. The path to understanding this process was stimulated at the start of the nineteenth century with the discovery that the body produced its own chemical substances, such as hydrochloric acid in the stomach, and iron in the blood. Research began to discover why these substances were present and to establish normal limits within the body. This would in turn help to diagnose discrepancies suggesting ill health. Additionally, these studies help to advance applicable treatments.

Physicians in Paris concluded that advancement by the use of dissection and patient examination could go no further. They decided that animal testing in the laboratory was a better option, as the study of human subjects was limited (Wootton 2006). This resulted in little advancement in experimental knowledge due to the differences in animal and human physiology.

William Prout (1785–1850) was a British chemical physiologist who recognised the inability to translate chemical processes in animals to human anatomy, and this led him to become a chemist. He carried out many experiments; most importantly in the field of diabetes, Prout studied human metabolism, and for 4 years from 1816, compared blood and urine, identifying the substance urea as a by-product of the kidneys (Prout 1821).

Prout's findings were published as *An Inquiry into the Treatment of Diabetes, Calculus and Other Affections*, being recognised as the standard text of the time on diseases of the stomach and kidneys. In 1827, his experiments showed the processes involved in human digestion and how carbohydrates are broken down into glucose. Prout was one of the first scientists to use biochemistry in the study of disease (Brock 1992).

Using animal experimentation for research purposes did have its problems, however, as often repeat experimentation produced no new results. This brought into force the 1876 Cruelty to Animals Act, meaning that animal research needed a licence issued by the Home Secretary (Wootton 2006).

The metabolic process was beginning to be understood. *Justus von Liebig* (1803–1873) was a German scientist who had come to the conclusion that oxygen in the lungs became mixed with starch for the digestion of carbohydrates. This energy was then taken up by the muscles, while waste was excreted in the urine. Von Liebig was able to measure with chemical analysis how much food and oxygen were taken in and how much energy was expelled (Brock 2002). However, most of his research was based on animal studies (Sheenstone 2009). These results were criticised by William Prout, who disputed the findings on the changing state of organic compounds in animals, which was later termed 'the intermediary metabolism'—complex biochemical reactions within body cells (Brock 1992). The work of von Liebig and Prout later became the science of biochemistry (Porter 2003).

Claude Bernard (1813–1878) was a French physiologist. The earlier work of John Rollo led diabetes to be seen as an abnormality of carbohydrate metabolism causing increased glucose to be absorbed in the gastrointestinal tract, following many experiments in 1855 exploring this subject in animals. Bernard declared that without vivisection, neither 'physiology nor scientific medicine is possible' (Wootton 2006). In 1857, Bernard discovered a secretion from the liver of animals that alters blood glucose levels. He documented this important finding, describing the conversion of excess glucose into glycogen by the liver to be stored (Bernard 1999).

We now know that the liver releases glucose into the bloodstream once a meal has been fully digested. If insulin is unable to work correctly in untreated type 2 diabetes, or barely present at all in untreated type 1 diabetes, blood glucose concentration rises, leading to high glucose levels.

Bernard proposed that diabetes must result from an alteration in glucose metabolism, since those with the disease had glucose in both their blood and urine. Bernard's chemical analysis showed how pancreatic secretions break down starch and proteins during digestion (Bernard 1999). The discipline of endocrinology—the study of the endocrine system and disorders of the endocrine glands—arose from these groundbreaking discoveries.

The Mystery of the Pancreas

The pancreas was first recognised as a distinct organ by Greek anatomist Herophilus in 300 B.C. While its anatomical structure was noted, the function of the pancreas, particularly its role in digestion and diabetes, was not fully understood for centuries. Autopsies had mainly been performed to determine the cause of death, noting any abnormalities in a particular organ.

The understanding that each organ in the body has a specific function developed gradually over centuries, with knowledge added by ancient Greek philosophers and physicians, as well as advancements in anatomy during the Renaissance. While the ancients recognised some organ functions, detailed knowledge and the study of body systems advanced significantly with the work of sixteenth-century anatomists like Andreas Vesalius.

Historically, it was observed during post-mortem examinations that there is change in the anatomical structure of the pancreas in people with diabetes. *Thomas Cawley* performed an autopsy on an individual who had died of diabetes; the anatomist was the first to report in 1788 that the pancreas appeared 'somewhat shrivelled, with tissue damage and the presence of stones in the pancreatic ducts' (Cawley 1788). However, no direct link between diabetes and the pancreas was immediately identified.

The Role of the Pancreas

We now know that the pancreas is both an endocrine and an exocrine gland. As an endocrine gland, it secretes hormones directly into the bloodstream, rather than through a duct; as an exocrine gland, it secretes digestive enzymes into the small intestine.

In the late eighteenth century, despite observable shrivelling of the pancreas, the function of the organ was yet to be determined. The search was on to discover how the pancreas was linked to diabetes. The role of the pancreas was finally discovered through a combination of anatomical studies, experiments on digestion and the eventual understanding of its endocrine function, particularly in regulating blood glucose levels. The pancreas had been previously regarded as a non-vital organ, involved in 'breaking down fatty matter and converting starch in the diet into sugar'.

Richard Bright (1789–1858) documented eight case reports in 1832 regarding the excretion of fat in the stools, but did not link this observation to diabetes, even when a patient with a diseased pancreas was seen at post-mortem. He stated: 'There is no connection between the two diseased actions' (Bright 1983). Bright made this conclusion based on having seen many patients with diabetes who did not have pale and fatty stools (Bright 1832).

There is now a recognised link between diabetes, gastrointestinal complications of diabetes affecting absorption, and excretion of fat in the stools (Murray and Emmanuel 2006).

The mystery of the pancreas and the role of the kidneys remained confused due to the condition of these organs at post-mortem. There was still a belief that the kidneys were glands, therefore having an unknown link with the pancreas. Without any clear physical sign of an association between diabetes and the kidneys researchers grew weary with the search, as can be seen below (Wilson 1847):

> Examination of the dead body throws little or no light upon the pathology of diabetes. We naturally look with interest to the kidneys. But we find nothing there to explain the symptoms noticed during life. I have noticed the deep purplish colour of the kidneys which were veined and vascular, but not otherwise altered in texture. Others tell us that the kidneys are found hypertrophied [excessively large] in diabetes. But hypertrophy and unnatural vascularity are circumstances which we are not surprised at when we reflect upon the vastly increased quantity of work which the glands [kidneys] have been performing. They are the consequences rather than the cause of the morbid flow of urine.

An increased blood supply within the kidneys in cases of diabetes was often seen at post-mortem, with reports stating that the organs were 'rather fuller of blood than usual, often enlarged and soft' (Eberle 1831). As far back as the fifth century A.D., Oribasius had noted that diseased kidneys accompanied those who had 'suffered excessive urination and thirst', describing the kidneys as hardened at post-mortem.

Paul Ehrlich (1854–1915) was the first to report that complications of diabetes are a direct result of long-term high blood glucose levels, the presence of abnormally increased levels of glucose in the blood being the direct cause of diabetic nephropathy (kidney disease). He showed that over months and years, high levels of glucose in the blood alters the structure of cells that line the kidney tubes, which are responsible for filtering waste and regulating fluid balance (Silverstein 2001).

In 1868, a medical student named *Paul Langerhans* published his findings on 'pancreatic islands' (Islam 2000). He identified that the pancreas contained distinct cells, one secreting pancreatic juices that we know are enzymes, while the other secreted 'an unknown substance'. These pancreatic islands are now known to be islet cells, secreting insulin. Langerhans found islet cells in his tissue samples, but thought they were lymph glands. Despite this oversight the islets were finally recognised as the insulin-producing cells of the pancreas.

Laguese, a French scientist, named the cells discovered by Langerhans 'the islets of Langerhans' after the medical student. Laguese had observed that the islet cells and the size of the pancreas shrank if the pancreatic duct in dogs was tied off. The function of the islets of Langerhans was determined by Laguese, advancing Langerhans' discovery further by observing minute structural changes in the insulin-producing cells of patients with diabetes (Islam 2000). This was also recognised by *Opie* in 1873, when he noted that the islet cells of a girl who had died from diabetes were in an advanced state of degeneration.

These were important milestones, but the significance was missed. There was no recognition of missing insulin as the key factor in type 1 diabetes, or the inability for insulin to work correctly in type 2 diabetes.

Inflammation of the pancreas that occurs in the condition pancreatitis was observed by German physiologist *Friedrich* in 1878, who found that excessive alcoholism could lead to this inflammation.

This condition is caused by pancreatic enzymes breaking down the pancreatic tissue (Prime 1987). Short-term (acute) pancreatitis is a severe and life-threatening condition; long-term (chronic) pancreatitis drastically disrupts the shape and function of the pancreas, which can cause type 1 diabetes.

Reginald Fitz was a pathologist who documented the clinical characteristics of pancreatitis while working at Harvard. Fitz observed that when the pancreas became severely inflamed, it 'filled with pus and blood and turned gangrenous, causing damage to the minute structures of the organ' (Murray 1969).

Oskar Minowski and *Joseph von Mering* were scientists trying to crack the cause of diabetes, and repeated Conrad Brunner's earlier experiments. Minowski and von Mering took this further and recognised that they had induced diabetes in dogs by removing the pancreas. The animals developed an 'unquenchable thirst and frequent urination' after several days. This was seen to be similar to people with diabetes. The dogs' urine showed high levels of glucose, hinting that the pancreas played a major role in the body (Medvei 1993). Despite this breakthrough, there was uncertainty over whether pancreatic secretions regulated blood glucose levels, or if this was a function of the kidneys.

As early as 752 A.D., when Chinese physician Wang Tao advocated feeding pork pancreas to people with diabetes, it yet again became a prominent treatment for diabetes in 1899. However, the consumption of pancreatic extracts did not reduce blood glucose levels as hoped because the extracts were broken down in the stomach, destroying any insulin. This is why insulin cannot be taken by mouth.

Giulio Vassale (1862–1913) was an Italian pathologist and pioneer of endocrinology who discovered that the destruction of the islet cells resulted in the non-production of pancreatic enzymes, proclaiming: 'the islets are the seat of the morbid process'. This knowledge was valuable in furthering the understanding of diabetes and the pancreas.

Massiglia confirmed the previous findings, suggesting that secretions from the islet cells governed carbohydrate metabolism, given the rise in blood and urinary glucose in people with diabetes after eating (Marwood 1973).

Ivan Petrovich Pavlov (1849–1936) was a Russian physiologist, best known for his work on conditioned reflexes that won him a Nobel Prize in 1904. His experiments with dogs included introducing acids into the duodenal glands; this stimulated the production of pancreatic secretions, confirming that duodenal secretions are controlled by the nervous system. Pavlov's *The Work of the Digestive Glands* was published in 1897, arising from lectures he had given on physiology (Pavlov 1910).

It was later realised why the deficit of insulin in untreated type 1 diabetes leads to ketoacidosis and diabetic coma—during insulin deficit, the body breaks down fat and protein for energy, instead of glucose. *Bernard Naunyn* (mentioned earlier for imprisoning diabetic patients so they could obtain 'sugar freedom') first used the term 'acidosis' to describe an abnormal accumulation of acids in the body.

Adolph Kussmaul was an endocrinologist who established ketoacidosis as the expression of a profound metabolic disorder in 1874; he described the 'great loud breathing' where the patient tries to pant these acids out of the body: 'the lungs heaved desperately to expel carbonic acid; the dying diabetic took huge gasps of air to increase his lung capacity' (Bliss 1988). Physicians termed this 'air hunger', likened to 'internal suffocation' (Murray 1969). Kussmaul showed that acid by-products known as ketone bodies (often smelling like pear drops, or nail varnish remover on the breath) can be seen in both the blood and urine. Severe ketoacidosis is a medical emergency, and Kussmaul breathing can precede death (Loriaux 2010).

The Nineteenth Century

At the beginning of the nineteenth century physicians attempted to treat diabetic coma. They did so by injecting sodium bicarbonate—an alkali—to neutralise the fatty acids. This 'proved largely ineffective in newly comatose patients, and never in cases of severe ketoacidosis and deep coma' (Bliss 1988).

Although formation of acids is a normal physiological process, *Magnus Levy* (1865–1955), together with Bernard Naunyn, suggested that inefficient use of carbohydrates in the lack of insulin prevents fats from being broken down in the usual way, resulting in the formation of fatty acids (Folin 1907). Rosenfeld had observed that 'fats burn in the flame of carbohydrates' (Pigman and Wolfrom 1968).

We now know that when insulin is in short supply, or not being produced at all, this causes the breakdown of muscle tissue and triglycerides—the most common type of fat found in the body and bloodstream, to use as fuel instead of glucose.

Towards the end of the nineteenth century there had been several attempts to cure diabetes. Despite a number of experiments demonstrating a clear connection between the pancreas and insulin deficit, advances in the understanding of diabetes reached a standstill.

- A 10-year-old child diagnosed with type 1 diabetes in 1897 had an average life expectancy of just 1.3 years.
- A 30-year-old adult developing type 2 diabetes at this time lived for an average of 4.1 years.
- A 50-year-old developing type 2 diabetes was expected to live for a total of 12 years because the disease began later in life (Allen 1915).

Because people with type 2 diabetes produce insulin, although it cannot work correctly if there is a high percentage of body fat impeding its action, the amount of insulin increases life expectancy in comparison with type 1 diabetes.

Summary

The newly established discipline of modern science was centred on chemistry by the end of the nineteenth century. The symptoms of diabetes were observed diagnostically, chemically analysed and accurately measured in order to characterise common and important factors. Scientific methods determined that excessive glucose seen in the blood and urine of people with diabetes had a connection with the pancreas; this was proved beyond doubt when removal of the organ in dogs resulted in extreme thirst and frequent urination. When tested, the insulin-producing islet cells of the pancreas appeared altered under the microscope.

This recognition allowed diabetes to be confirmed as a disorder of the digestive system; scientific research then returned to the importance of balanced nutrition and dietary management of type 2 diabetes. As we are seeing today, type 2 diabetes was far more common than the rarer type 1 diabetes. The discovery and availability of an effective glucose-lowering treatment for type 1 diabetes could not come soon enough for patients, although this miracle of medicine would take several more decades.

References

Allen FM (1915) The treatment of diabetes. Boston Med Surg J 172:241–247

Bernard C (1999) Experimental medicine. Transaction Publishers, Piscataway

Bliss M (1988) The discovery of insulin. Faber and Faber Limited, London

Bright R (1832) Causes and observations connected with disease of the pancreas and duodenum (Medico-chirurgical transactions). London: Longman, Rees, Orme, Brown, Green and Longman

Bright, P. (1983) Dr. Richard Bright (1789–1858). London: The Bodley Head Limited

Brock WH (1992) The Fontana history of chemistry. Fontana Press, Harper Collins Publishing, London

Brock WH (2002) Justus von Liebig: the chemical gatekeeper. Cambridge University Press, Cambridge

Cawley T (1788) A single case of diabetes, consisting entirely in the quality of urine; with observation into the different theories of the disease. Lond Med J 9:286–308

Dobson M (1776) Experiments and observations on the urine in diabetes. Med Observ Inq 5:298–310

Eberle J (1831) Treatise on the practice of medicine. John Grigg, Philadelphia

Folin O (1907) The acid intoxication theory. J Am Med Assoc XLIX(2):128–131

Islam S (2000) The islets of Langerhans. Springer, New York

Loriaux DL (2010) Adolph Kussmaul (1822–1902): the endocrinologist. Endocrinol Diabetes Obes 20(3):95

Marwood SF (1973) Diabetes mellitus – some reflections. J R Coll Gen Pract 23:38

Medvei VX (1993) The history of clinical endocrinology. The Parthenon Publishing Group Incorporated, New York

Miller, F.P, Vandrome, A.F., McBrewster, J. (ed.) (2010) Moritz Traube: Justus von Liebig, Louis Pasteur, Felix Hoppe-Seyler, Justus von Sachs, Ludwig Traube (physician), William Traube, Herman Traube. Beau Bassin: Alphascript Publications

Morgan M (2004) The evolution of the nutritional management of diabetes. Proc Nutr Soc 63:615–620

Murray I (1969) The search for insulin. Scott Med J 14:286–293

Murray C, Emmanuel A (2006) Chapter 8: Diabetes: chronic complications. In: Diabetes and the gastrointestinal system, 2nd edn. Wiley, Chichester

Pavlov IP (1910) The work of the digestive glands, Second English edition. Charles Griffin, London

Pavy F (1862) Researches on the nature and treatment of diabetes. Part 1: on the detection of sugar – qualitative and quantitative analysis. T. Gillet, London

Pavy FW (2009) The physiology of the carbohydrates. Their application as food and relation to diabetes. Read Books, London

Pigman WW, Wolfrom ML (1968) Advances in carbohydrates chemistry. Elsevier, Academic, Maryland Heights

Porter R (2003) Blood and guts: a short history of medicine. Penguin Books Limited, London

Prime N (1987) Introduction to pathology for radiographers. Butler and Tanner Limited, Frome/London

Prout, W. (1821) An inquiry into the nature and treatment of gravel, calculus, and other diseases. London. Second edition re-titled Inquiry into the treatment of diabetes, calculus and other affections, London, 1835. Third edition re-titled On the nature and treatment of stomach and urinary diseases, London, 1840. Fourth edition re-titled On the nature and treatment of stomach and renal diseases, London, 1843. Fifth edition, London, 1848

Rollo J (1797) An account of two cases of diabetes mellitus with remarks as they arose during the progress of the cure. T. Gillet, London

Sheenstone WA (2009) Justus von Liebig: his life and work (1803–1873). Bibliobazaar/Bibliolife, Charleston

Silverstein AM (2001) Paul Ehrlich's receptor immunology: the magnificent obsession. Academic Press, San Diego

Wheeler ML (2003) Cycles: diabetes nutrition recommendations – past, present and future. Diabetes Spectrum 13(3):116–119

Wilson T (1847) Principles and practice of physic. Lea and Blanchard, Philadelphia

Withers CWJ, Wood P (eds) (2002) Science and medicine in the Scottish enlightenment. Tuckwell Press Limited, East Linton

Wootton D (2006) Bad medicine: doctors doing harm since Hippocrates. Oxford University Press, New York

5

The Significance of Insulin

Since the time that diabetes was first recognised as a disease, there had always been a pressing need to discover a cure. Many ideas and treatments had been put forward, with little or no success, especially for type 1 diabetes. Chemical methods in 1900 made diabetes easy to diagnose, and urine could now be tested to show the level of glucose present; however, glucose levels could not be controlled (Allen 1913). In the same year, William Bayliss and Ernest Starling detected chemical messengers within the bloodstream that controlled secretions from the endocrine glands, and in 1902, suggested the term 'hormone' to describe any secretion from an endocrine gland.

With the final identification of the insulin-producing islet cells of the pancreas, discovered in 1869, a link had been established showing the process from consumption to digestion. Although pancreatic islet cell clusters had been recognised, further research was necessary to determine the function of this hormone in diabetes. The answers to these mysterious questions pushed research forward at a pace to find a treatment for type 1 diabetes.

A Host of Experiments

Eugene Lindsay Opie (1873–1971) was a pathology tutor at the Johns Hopkins University, who felt that there was a great deal of literature available on the subject of diabetes. In 1900–1901, he confirmed the association between marked deterioration of the islet cells and the onset of diabetes, and concluded that normal metabolism of glucose was only possible with pancreatic secretions (Opie 2009). However, this conclusion had already been established.

V. Wilson, *Diabetes Ancient and Modern*, Hippocrates,
https://doi.org/10.1007/978-3-032-12454-8_5

Sobolev (Ssobelow) and *Schulze* carried out pancreatic research in Germany at the beginning of the twentieth century, using a technique known as ligation to prevent the pancreatic duct in dogs from secreting enzymes. This repeated similar research and showed in the same way that the pancreas became contracted with tissue wasting, although the islet cells were unaffected, and the animals did not have diabetes as a result (Rosenfeld 2002).

Similarly, *Moses Barron* showed that the islet cells were unaffected by the presence of pancreatic stones in the two human pancreatic ducts, concluding that the patient had no diabetes symptoms (Barron 1920).

Although this had been tried orally as a treatment, with the result that the extract was broken down in the patient's digestive process, pancreatic extracts had not previously been administered both orally *and* injected in the same experiment. To observe any outcome, *John Rennie* and *Thomas Fraser* experimented by injecting five patients with islet extracts from 1902 to 1904. This was obtained from the pancreatic tissues of fish and snakes, where it was seen to 'form separate globular aggregates' (Rennie and Fraser 1907). There was no change in the patient's raised blood glucose as a result.

Further work involving pancreatic tissue continued with *Jean de Meyer* (1878–1934), who highlighted the presence of a substance 'insuline', produced by the islet cells in 1904–1909 (De Meyer 1909). This term was the same as that used by Sharpey-Schäfer in 1913, although he denied all knowledge of de Meyer calling the substance insuline in 1909 (Rosenfeld 2002). The pancreas is a complex organ with multiple functions, and this made the chemical extraction of insulin problematic.

In 1908, *Georg Ludwig Zuelzer* prepared a pancreatic extract he termed 'acomatrol' and tested this on rabbits before injecting a patient who was near to death (Howard and Hess 2002). Although there was 'some improvement', there were no blood or urine tests, and the patient died a few days later (Murray 1969). Tests may not have been carried out due to the 10–20 mL of blood needed to perform a glucose test (Rosenfeld 2002). Zuelzer continued to inject five more patients with his impure extract, causing abscesses and a high temperature, although a pharmaceutical manufacturer eventually helped him to purify his discovery. In 1911, despite the earlier outcome, Zuelzer patented his extract as: 'Pancreas Preparation Suitable for the Treatment of Diabetes' (Murray 1969).

The search for the elusive pancreatic secretion that controlled blood glucose sparked researchers to experiment with pancreatic extracts. *Ernest Lyman Scott* (1877–1966) followed in the footsteps of Minowski and von Mering to find a pancreatic extract that reduced blood glucose when injected. Scott conducted practical research with dogs in the same way, seeing flies around the frequent puddles of urine that were passed, concluding that the urine must contain glucose (Scott 1912).

Taking the work of Minowski and von Mering further—who were not fully certain of the role of pancreatic secretions—Scott saw that glucose levels in dogs increased in the blood and urine following removal of the pancreas. Scott achieved a short-lived reduction in the dogs' glucose levels and urine production after injecting his isolated extract (Rosenfeld 2002). Despite this, he was reluctant to publish the results, believing the effect could be due to factors other than the extract: 'It does not follow that these effects are due to the internal secretion of the pancreas in the extract' (Scott 1913). Scott then gave up on what would have been the discovery of insulin, leaving his work behind in the laboratory (Murray 1969).

Although the degeneration of pancreatic islet cells in diabetes was well-established, these experiments were again repeated to ensure reliability and validity of results. As such, *Edward Sharpey-Schäfer* (1850–1935), a physiology professor at Edinburgh University, concluded that the pancreas was minus a single chemical in diabetes, identifying that the pancreatic islet cells potentially controlled glucose metabolism by secreting this missing chemical. Although actually a hormone, he named the chemical 'insuline' in 1913 (Sharpey-Schäfer 1914).

Just before the First World War, *Nicolas Paulesco* induced low glucose levels in dogs by injecting them with filtered sterile ground pancreas in water, named 'pancreatine' (Rosenfeld 2002). While trying to distil the extract further in Budapest, Paulesco held off from publishing these promising results until 1921. Meanwhile, at the same time in Canada, similar research has seen various publications regarding a groundbreaking discovery by Banting and Best.

The Most Significant Medical Discovery in History

Although the pancreas is a large organ, only about 1% of its cells constitute the islets of Langerhans, the area of the pancreas producing insulin (Tortora and Grabowski 1993). The term 'hormone', suggested by Bayliss and Starling in 1902 comes from the Greek meaning 'I set in motion'. Secretions from the endocrine system change certain body cells, and 'hormone' was then used to describe all secretions from the endocrine tissue (Bayliss and Starling 1902). The work of Sharpey-Schäfer made it clear that the pancreas breaks down carbohydrates which the body can then use in the form of glucose; a hormone then acted to control blood glucose levels (Sharpey-Schäfer 1914).

Frederick Banting (1891–1941) continued the work of Ernest Scott by attempting to isolate the pancreatic hormone as a treatment for type 1 diabetes. As a surgeon and not a research scientist, Banting was prompted to contact *John Macleod*, Professor of physiology at Toronto University. Macleod, however, believed diabetes that had been induced in dogs was due to elevated glucose from the liver, although he did give Banting research students, Charles Best (1899–1978) and Edward Noble (1900–1978), laboratory time and animal subjects (Bliss 1988).

Macleod's work added to the knowledge of glucose use by muscles, although he did not value the part played by pancreatic secretions on glucose levels (Macleod 1922). Macleod studied the outcome on depancreatised (removed) dogs, concluding that pancreatic secretions had a role in the glucose available for muscles to work (Macleod and Pearce 1913).

Banting and his research students were keen to experiment with human subjects with diabetes. They asked Macleod and research biochemist, James Collip, to work with them on the purification of the pancreatic extracts. They continued to experiment with dogs, managing to successfully treat those whose pancreases had been removed; their pancreatic extract was sourced from cattle. Repeating this success in humans with diabetes was the next step.

In December 1921, Banting and his research students, along with Collip, improved the quality of their extract, 'isletin' (Bliss 1988). The team's findings were presented at Yale University in the 34th annual meeting of the American Physiological Society. Collip and the team used their now-improved isletin on rabbits to ensure the substance was pure enough to avoid the formation of abscesses (Collip 1923).

The team continued their testing on dogs, stabilising the temperature of the insuline at 35 °C, the longest-surviving dog living for 70 days. The dog's glucose levels became stabilised with isletin injections, with no glucose seen in the urine. This was a major breakthrough, as previous subjects had only survived for 2 weeks (Banting and Best 1922a, b). Temperature control and evaporation, along with maintaining pH levels, were a major factor in their success.

On 4 August 1921, isletin was felt to be pure enough to use on human subjects (Bliss 1988). The discovery of isletin prompted many papers to be published, although there were no studies regarding any long-term effects in humans associated with the treatment of type 1 diabetes (Banting et al. 1922a, b, c, d, e).

The First Human Subject

In January 1922, at Toronto General Hospital, Leonard Thompson—a 14-year-old boy—became the first to receive isletin. He was in the final stages of type 1 diabetes and near-death, weighing only 65 pounds (4 stone, 6 pounds) and with breath smelling of acetone (Rosenfeld 2002; Bliss 1988). He had been placed on a starvation diet, but with little hope of survival, making him the ideal test subject. His blood glucose level was 440 decilitres per litre (U.S. measurement), equivalent to 24.4 millilitres per litre (UK measurement). After the administration of isletin, his blood glucose level dropped over the next 24 hours to 320 dL/L (17.8 mmol/L) (Russell 2012).

Leonard Thompson was prescribed 85 units of isletin a day (Bliss 1988) and his diabetes was considered to be 'poorly controlled'. As an older teenager, he was able to work, although he did drink alcohol regularly (Bliss 1988). He was hospitalised once in a comatose state due to high blood glucose levels in 1932, and in 1935, at the age of 27, he developed pneumonia and died. The cause of his death, although due to infection, was the development of high blood glucose levels and ketoacidosis; infection increases the need for insulin by as much as three times the normal dosage (Laffel 2000), although this was not known at the time.

The Nobel Prize for Medicine was awarded for the discovery of insulin in October 1923, even though this was only a year after the first human test subject (Bliss 1988). However, due to Nobel Prize rules, everyone involved did not share in the accolade. Banting and Macleod received the award, even though Macleod was on holiday at the actual time of the discovery—receiving the award because the discovery had been made in his laboratory. Outraged, Banting shared half his prize money with Charles Best, while Macleod suggested he would share half of his money with James Collip.

The Nobel Committee later admitted that Best should have shared the Prize with Banting (Rosenfeld 2002). Despite this oversight, Banting and Best are jointly credited with the discovery of insulin in 1921.

The Production of Insulin

Derived from the Latin for 'island', the word 'insulin' was suggested by Professor John Macleod (Bliss 1988). The name 'isletin' became 'insulin' because the latter was uncontaminated and isolated from the whole pancreas, rather than extracts (Rosenfeld 2002).

Following the success with Leonard Thompson shortly after the production of pure insulin in 1922, a further high-profile case showed the miracle of insulin, where an emaciated young girl regained her health, ultimately living to the age of 73 (Cooper and Ainsberg 2010). Similarly in Edinburgh, Purvis Walker—Treasurer of the Royal College of Surgeons—grew very thin and extremely weak and near death, having endured untreated type 1 diabetes for 2 years. He was sent some insulin by Banting, although Walker actually gave it to a young boy, considering his need to be greater. Walker also received insulin treatment before it was commercially available, his doctor recording the almost instant reduction in his blood glucose (Murray 1969):

> This saved his life. The transformation was nothing short of marvelous and in a few weeks, he had put on several stones in weight and looked as he had done before his illness.

The first Diabetes Department was formed at the Edinburgh Royal Infirmary, using insulin produced by J.C. Meakins, the first company to do so in 1923. Over 40 years later, Sir Derrick Dunlop, Professor of Therapeutics and Clinical Medicine, commented that insulin treatment was 'unique because it gave maximum relief with minimum effort', adding (Dunlop 1966):

> I have never seen anything in medicine more heart-warming or rewarding than to watch those diabetic patients raise themselves step by step out of the valley of the shadow of death.

The patent for insulin was held by J.C. Macleod in Toronto, Canada. He agreed insulin could be produced by J.C. Meakins in the UK, allowing the UK Medical Research Council the patent through his friend, Sir Henry Dale. Insulin was eventually available in units, a measurement to allow a consistent dosage (Sinding 2002). A major advance in insulin production occurred when the manufacture of sterile cow (bovine) insulin began by American pharmaceutical giant, Eli Lilly in May 1922 (Murray 1969). In 1923 The Nordisk Insulin Company teamed up with Novo, making Denmark the second most prominent country outside America to produce insulin (Rosenfeld 2002).

Not All Plain Sailing

Insulin was initially only available to patients for purchase. Chemists sold insulin in powdered form, and this had to be fully dissolved in boiling water and cooled before injection. This frequently caused inflammation and chambers of pus to form at the injection site. Despite this disadvantage, the improvement in health was worth it. Figures from the New York Metropolitan Life Assurance Company show that between 1899 and 1914, deaths from high glucose causing diabetic coma totalled 65% (Marwood 1973). Following the discovery of insulin, this fell to 15% in 1923 for people with type 1 diabetes.

Inequalities existed for those who could not afford to buy their insulin, while some physicians were slow to accept the new wonder drug (Bliss 1988). Nothing has changed regarding the inaccessibility of insulin in poorer countries, where insulin is not consistently available, and types of insulin vary greatly.

The subject of patients not doing what they are told to by their physician has always been a barrier to good health with diabetes. Sometimes, the availability of insulin was and still is misused, forcing The Metropolitan Life Assurance Company to issue a warning in 1926:

> Occasionally a patient under insulin treatment feels so much better that he is tempted to abandon his diet and eat everything he wants. But when he does, he is likely to suffer a relapse and die. Then insulin is blamed.

In 1927, Elliot Joslin stated that a diabetes regime was not often adhered to, with patients often 'failing to achieve this optimal dietary treatment'. He suggested that all patients with diabetes should eat a 'weighed' diet comprising 22% carbohydrates, 16% fats and 62% proteins, although in his opinion, (Joslin 1927):

> Many children and a few adults have not yet reached this quantity of carbohydrates [meaning 22 percent daily intake], but I recall none who are now taking less than 50 grams. Furthermore, one can observe a steady increase in this amount, formerly considered liberal.

During the late 1920s, following the discovery of insulin and this new diabetes regime that could easily make a patient unconscious with low blood glucose, patients often made mistakes. Fifty years later saw the tables turn from Joslin's theory, and patients with type 1 diabetes were required to eat a high-carbohydrate diet to balance the amount of insulin they had injected.

Historical Advances in Diabetes Treatment

1922: Insulin was first produced to work at different rates, to match the body's own insulin requirements. The first two short-acting insulins to be produced were 'quick-acting' (soluble) and 'fast-acting' (regular) (Marwood 1973). This required two to four injections per day.

1934: The British Diabetic Association was founded by author H.G. Wells and scientist R.D. Lawrence, who both had type 2 diabetes.

1935: Nordisk introduced Protamine zinc insulin (a fish protein) with a delayed working time (Marwood 1973). The effect of more flexible insulin regimes can be seen in the 1941 comment below from the Metropolitan Life Assurance Company (Marwood 1973):

> The diabetic whose disease is discovered early; who promptly puts himself under and stays under his physician's guidance; and who masters the details of his treatment, stands a good chance of living as long as he could reasonably expect to live without diabetes.

1938: Dr. Alexis Carrel experimented with transplantation of animal pancreases in the search for a cure for diabetes. In the same year, the speedy recovery from hypoglycaemia following administration of glucose was described by Allen Whipple (Johna and Schein 2003).

1940: Allen Whipple removed a pancreatic islet cell tumour from a patient. In the same year, Professor Sir Hans Krebs described the metabolic process leading to diabetes (Holmes 1994).

1944: Everest introduced the standardised stainless steel and glass insulin syringe.

1945: Isophane neutral (Insulatard) insulin was developed with an extended working time, especially when combined with regular insulin to cover the rise in blood glucose after eating.

1953: Novo introduced Lente, Ultralente and Semilente insulins to better match the patient's daily routine (Pyke 1997). These proved popular, and one third of people worldwide were taking this form of insulin (Marwood 1973).

1957: The drug laboratory at Boots the Chemist was one of three leading UK insulin manufacturers.

1961: Becton Dickinson introduced the disposable plastic insulin syringe.

1966: An effective and complete transplant of the pancreas was achieved at Manitoba University Hospital.

1969: Ames Diagnostics introduced the first portable blood glucose meter for use in hospitals. This was developed in 1971 for patients to use in their own homes (Bernstein 2011).

1973: Novo introduced Monocomponent (MC) ultra-pure insulin (Pyke 1997).

1981: Transplantation as a treatment for type 1 diabetes was suggested by Patrick J. Broe.

1982: Eli Lilly and Company formed a 'human insulin' solution using DNA technology. In the same year, Human Monocomponent pig insulin was introduced by Novo that matches the action of human insulin (Pyke 1997).

1986: Novo introduced the insulin pen.

1987: Novo began to genetically manufactured insulin from yeast to avoid the use of animal pancreases.

1996: Lilly introduced insulin Lispro, known as Humalog, with a short acting time to be injected after a meal.

1997: Dr. Richard Bernstein buys his own glucose meter and maintains good diabetes control for over 40 years. His book (now in its fourth edition) recognises this link and guides patients on how to avoid the development of diabetic complications with good glucose control (Bernstein 2011).

2000: Lantus insulin was introduced in the U.S. It works for 24 hours and has a continual acting time without peaks.

2003: Insulin pumps were first used in research in the 1970s and 1980s. Mode pumps became smaller and user-friendly in the early 2000s.

2004: Pfizer, Aventis and Nektar Therapeutics, introduced their insulin inhaler, where insulin is drawn into the lungs as a fine powder (NICE 2006; Rosenstock et al. 2004). This was approved in the UK for type 1 and type 2 diabetes in 2006.

Summary

In the early twentieth century most doctors thought that diabetes was more severe if the patient had fewer islet cells working, and that high blood glucose levels over-taxed the remaining functional cells. Starvation diets were prescribed to control the effects of insulin deficit; it was hoped that lower blood glucose levels would allow the islet cells to rest and regenerate, restoring the individual to normal health. This led to malnutrition in many patients with type 1 diabetes, who then caught an infection and died.

Insulin is undoubtedly the most important medical discovery in history. Having seen the improvement in symptoms following a starvation diet, it followed that insulin injections would allow the islets to regain normal function and begin to produce insulin once more. Only later was it realised that the islet cells are continually destroyed by the patient's immune system in type 1 diabetes.

Many other advances in the treatment of diabetes and the recognition of how the disease affects the body have been made since these momentous treatment discoveries. However, the battle to keep blood glucose levels normal in an effort to prevent or reduce the occurrence of chronic complications remains a major problem for people with diabetes, and for the health professionals providing their care. This is because diabetes may be very difficult to control effectively for proactive patients, and overwhelmingly, because many people in the diabetes population show a lack of motivation for diabetes self-management to prevent further serious health problems.

References

Allen FM (1913) Studies concerning glycosuria and diabetes. Harvard University Press, Cambridge, MA

Banting FG, Best CH (1922a) The internal secretion of the pancreas. J Lab Clin Med 7:251–266

Banting FG, Best CH (1922b) The internal secretions of the pancreas. J Lab Clin Med 7:251–266

Banting FG, Best CH, Macleod JJR (1922a) The internal secretions of the pancreas (Abstract). Am J Physiol 59:479

Banting FG, Best CH, Collip JK et al (1922b) Pancreatic extracts in the treatment of diabetes mellitus. J Can Med Assoc 12:141–146

Banting FG, Best CH, Collip JK et al (1922c) The effects of insulin on experimental hyperglycaemia in rabbits. Am J Physiol 62:559–580

Banting FG, Best CH, Collip JK et al (1922d) Pancreas extracts in the treatment of diabetes mellitus. Preliminary report. Can Med Assoc J 12:141–146

Banting FG, Best CH, Collip JK et al (1922e) The effect produced on diabetes by extracts of the pancreas. Assoc Am Physicians 37:337–347

Barron M (1920) The relation of the islets of Langerhans to diabetes with special reference to pancreatic lithiasis. Surg Gynecol Obstet 31:437–448

Bayliss WM, Starling EH (1902) The mechanism of pancreatic secretion. J Physiol 28:325–353

Bernstein R (2011) Dr. Bernstein's diabetes solutions: the complete guide to achieving normal blood sugars, 4th edn. Little Brown & Company, New York

Bliss M (1988) The discovery of insulin. Faber and Faber, London

Collip JB (1923) The history of the discovery of insulin. Northwest Med 22:267–273

Cooper T, Ainsberg A (2010) Breakthrough: Elizabeth Hughes, the discovery of insulin, and the making of a medical miracle. MacMillan/St. Martin's Press, New York

De Meyer J (1909) Actions of the internal secretions of the pancreas on different organs and kidney secretions. Arch Physiol 7:96–99

Dunlop DD (1966) Opening address for "diabetes mellitus", symposium of the University of Edinburgh, Pfizer Foundation for post-graduate medical research. University of Edinburgh, Pfizer Monographs 1:1–6

Holmes FL (1994) Hans Krebs: architect of intermediary metabolism, 1933–1937. Open University Press, New York

Howard JM, Hess W (2002) A history of the pancreas: mysteries of a hidden organ. Springer, New York

Johna S, Schein M (2003) The memoirs of Allen Oldfather Whipple: the man behind the Whipple operation. TFM Publishing Limited, Wiltshire

Joslin EP (1927) The diabetic diet. J Am Diet Assoc 3:89–92

Laffel L (2000) Sick-day management in type 1 diabetes. Endocrinol Metab Clin N Am 29(4):707–723

Macleod JJR (1922) The source of insulin. A study of the effect produced on blood sugar by the pancreas and principal islets of fishes. J Metab Res 2:149–172

Macleod JJR, Pearce RG (1913) The sugar consumption in normal and diabetic (depancreatised) dogs after evisceration. Am J Physiol 32:184–199

Marwood SF (1973) Diabetes mellitus—some reflections. J R Coll Gen Practit 23:38–45

Murray I (1969) The search for insulin. Scott Med J 14:286–293

National Institute for Health and Clinical Excellence (2006) Appraisal of inhaled insulin for diabetes (type 1 and type 2). National Institute for Health and Clinical Excellence, London

Opie EL (2009) Disease of the pancreas: its cause and nature. General Books LLC, Memphis

Pyke DA (1997) The history of diabetes. In: Alberti KGMM, Zimmet P, DeFronzo RA (eds) International textbook of diabetes mellitus, 2nd edn. Wiley, London

Rennie J, Fraser T (1907) The Islets of Langerhans in relation to diabetes. J Biochem 2:7–19

Rosenfeld L (2002) Insulin: discovery and controversy. Clin Chem 48(12):2270–2288

Rosenstock J, Cappelleri J, Bolinder B et al (2004) Patient satisfaction and glycaemic control after 1 year with inhaled insulin (Exubera) in patients with type 1 and type 2 diabetes. Diabetes Care 27:1318–1323

Russell RC (2012) Diabetic Ketoacidosis. VSD Publications, Seattle

Scott EL (1912) On the influence of intravenous injections of an extract of the pancreas on experimental diabetes. Am J Physiol 29:306–310

Scott EL (1913) The relation of pancreatic extract to the sugar of the blood. Soc Exp Biol Med 10:101–103

Sharpey-Schäfer E (1914) An introduction to the endocrine glands and internal secretions. Stanford University, Palo Alto

Sinding C (2002) Making the unit of insulin: standards, clinical work and industry, 1920–1925. Bull Hist Med 76(2):231–270

Tortora GJ, Grabowski SR (1993) Principles of anatomy and physiology, 7th edn. Harper Collins Publishers, New York

6

What of Type 2 Diabetes?

As we have seen throughout history, the number of people developing type 2 diabetes has steadily risen due to the increased availability and use of sugar in wealthier classes, which slowly filtered down to the lower classes. Dietary restrictions imposed during wartime food rationing showed that weight loss reduced glucose levels in patients with type 2 diabetes, proving the causal link between eating fewer carbohydrates and better diabetes control.

With the increased availability of food after the Second World War, and the resulting increase in carbohydrate intake as sugar rationing was lifted, cases of type 2 diabetes multiplied rapidly in association with the post-war 'sugar craze' (Offord 2024). There had always been a need for a treatment for type 2 diabetes to accompany a healthy diet and regular exercise. A chance discovery led to the development of a suitable treatment.

The Distinction Between Types of Diabetes

In the early twentieth century following the discovery of insulin, there was no classification to guide which patients required insulin treatment, and those who could control their diabetes with diet alone. Before a distinction between type 1 and type 2 diabetes was clearly made, there was no register of who was taking insulin and who was not. While a type of diabetes with less severe symptoms had been observed and recorded since ancient times, type 2 was not properly distinguished as different from type 1 diabetes until the 1930s.

V. Wilson, *Diabetes Ancient and Modern*, Hippocrates,
https://doi.org/10.1007/978-3-032-12454-8_6

In 1936, British diabetologist *Harold Himsworth*, first proposed that many patients were resistant to insulin, rather than having the insulin deficit associated with type 1 diabetes (Himsworth 1936).

We now know that *insulin resistance* (when cells in muscles, fat, and the liver don't respond well to insulin) is the crucial factor in the type 2 diabetes disease pathway; type 2 diabetes is a consequence of both insulin resistance and impairment of the insulin-producing cells (Cavaghan et al. 2000).

After carrying out further research by asking his patients questions, Himsworth determined that there were two different pathways to diabetes: a deficit of insulin in those with rapid onset of type 1 diabetes in their younger years (Krentz and Hitman 2011); and poor insulin sensitivity which had occurred over several years in older patients with type 2 diabetes. Despite this advance in understanding the two main types of diabetes, Himsworth found that many physicians were slow to accept these conclusions (Himsworth 2011).

Over several more years, research to determine the disease pathways in diabetes showed that the vast majority—up to 95%—of diabetes is due to insulin insensitivity, and is therefore type 2; the remaining 5% of diabetes is the rarer type 1, due to insulin deficit (Krentz and Hitman 2011). This research proved Himsworth to be correct.

Further theories emerged to explain the difference between the individual causes of type 1 and type 2 diabetes. In the 1950s biologist, *Arthur Mirsky* proposed that the insulin produced by patients with type 2 diabetes was almost immediately broken down by enzymes so it could not work correctly (Pyke 1997).

In 1960, *Rosalyn Yalow* and *Solomon Berson* used radioactive insulin to investigate Mirsky's theory in people with type 2 diabetes, and in those who did not have type 2. Mirsky's theory of enzyme destruction in type 2 diabetes was shown to be incorrect, as the radioactive insulin was absorbed at a slower rate and was not quickly broken down by enzymes. Insulin insensitivity was again shown to be the most likely cause of type 2 diabetes. We now know that the insulin-producing cells of the pancreas eventually become weaker over time, resulting in what is known as insulin resistance (Kroker et al. 2008).

A Breakthrough in Treating Type 2?

In 1918, patients who had their parathyroid gland removed were shown to have an increase of a chemical compound—guanidine—in their bloodstream. This chemical, which is produced by the body as a normal part of protein metabolism, appeared to lower blood glucose levels, and researchers began animal studies with guanidine as a potential treatment for type 2 diabetes (Marwood 1973). However, guanidine itself was found to be toxic (Bailey 2017).

Throughout history, both type 1 and type 2 diabetes have been treated with restrictive diets as the only course of action. Before the discovery of insulin, diabetes specialist Dr. *Frederick Allen* wrote *Total Dietary Regulations in the Treatment of Diabetes* (Allen 1919). Without the distinction between types of diabetes, Allen treated both conditions with a very low-calorie diet and limited activity, which helped patients with type 2 diabetes. However, this was not sustainable, and patients were not eating a nutritious diet, lowering their immunity against infection (Pyke 1997).

As diabetes research progressed towards a cure, textbooks on the condition were written by *John Macleod* (Macleod 1913), who would later be associated with the discovery of insulin at Toronto University, and Dr. *Elliot Joslin* (Joslin 1927). As an expert in managing what would later be known as type 2 diabetes with diet and exercise, Joslin had seen the number of deaths from diabetes steadily increasing; consequently, Joslin felt that strict adherence to a diet and exercise regime was the only way patients could manage their condition. Diabetes medicine benefitted greatly from the five decades of his life that Joslin devoted to finding a cure.

In the 1920s and 1930s, the plant goat's rue was found to contain the chemical guanidine and its by-products (known as biguanides), including a substance called metformin. Excluding metformin as a weaker biguanide, these were used to treat high glucose levels, although this fizzled out with the knowledge of toxicity and as insulin became more widely available (Bailey 2017).

You may wonder why patients were not started on insulin treatment immediately after their diagnosis of type 2 diabetes. This is not the usual course of action because the condition can often be managed with lifestyle changes and oral medications. Treatment with insulin begins at a time when the initial oral medicines can no longer control levels of blood glucose.

The ability of biguanides to lower blood glucose—a group of diabetes drugs that work by reducing the amount of glucose produced by the liver—was advanced with the introduction of synthalin. In 1927, this had been synthesised by *Erich Frank* and colleagues in Germany (Schäfer 1983). 'Synthalin A' was available in tablet form and as a solution for injection. Although successful in reducing blood glucose in people with type 2 diabetes, it was eventually discovered that synthalin did not work as well in higher doses, and also raised serious concerns over associated liver and kidney damage, and some deaths (Bhattacharyya 2001).

Marcel Janbon, a French pharmacologist was working on a cure for typhoid in the 1940s, experimenting with extracts of French lilac (goat's rue). He stumbled upon the forgotten properties of the plant when the animal subjects in his research developed uncharacteristic behaviour, later found to be low blood glucose levels (Bhattacharyya 2001). Realising that guanidine stimulates the release of insulin, the possibilities for patients with type 2 diabetes not treated with insulin materialised. Janbon tested his theory, resulting in a drug called carbutamide following clinical trials with human subjects. Once again, while the effect of lowering blood glucose was achieved, the outcome of the drug was less advantageous, with research subjects suffering jaundice, gastric problems and death in some cases (Hermann 1979; Marwood 1973).

In 1957 *Jean Sterne* used metformin successfully to treat diabetes, despite the fact that it had been previously used to treat malaria in the 1940s (Hadden 2005). Metformin, containing two linked molecules of guanidine, was found to be non-toxic.

Following his experiments, Sterne (1957) wrote:

> Metformin is…well tolerated, which, even after very prolonged administration, does not damage the organism. At low doses, it is hypoglycaemic by mouth in the rabbit, chicken, rat, guinea pig, dog, alloxan-diabetic rabbit [experimentally created diabetes], and the diabetic human…and its ultimate place in the management of diabetes requires further study. (Bailey 2017)

Now a widely prescribed biguanide, metformin was not always well received as it was felt that it worked less well than other biguanides. Two of these—phenformin and buformin—were mostly discontinued in the late 1970s due to a high chance of dangerous lactic acid build-up in the bloodstream (Pillans 1998).

A Different Type of Diabetes Drug

When a patient has type 2 diabetes, their body develops insulin resistance, where body cells cannot respond normally to insulin. The pancreas begins to produce more and more insulin to try and reduce blood glucose levels, although this cannot be sustained. Eventually, glucose levels rise, resulting in type 2 diabetes.

A group of medicines known as sulfonamides proved effective in delaying this over-production of insulin and the resulting degeneration of the islet cells for several years. These medicines had the advantage of delaying the need to take insulin, but every year saw a 10% reduction in the ability to reduce blood glucose levels (Bhattacharyya 2001).

Sulfonylureas were first introduced for the treatment of type 2 diabetes in the 1950s: Tolbutamide was a far safer medicine for type 2 diabetes, introduced by Dr. *H. N. Halse*. Sulfonylureas are a class of diabetes drugs that stimulate the pancreas to release more insulin. Although this is the case, there may still not be enough produced to counteract the insulin resistance seen in type 2 diabetes. A safe and effective insulin resistance medicine that would also lower blood glucose was needed.

When compared with drugs to increase the production of insulin, guanidine by-products were no longer as popular, given their side effects and reduced ability to lower blood glucose in animal studies (Shapiro et al. 1959; Beckmann 1971). The stronger form of metformin, known as phenformin initially had shown huge promise as an alternative, until dangerous side effects were recognised and the drug was withdrawn (McKendry et al. 1959; Butterfield 1968).

There seemed to be an uncertain outlook for metformin, despite the clear differences between other biguanides and sulfonylureas. By reducing glucose production in the liver, metformin helps control blood glucose, and improves insulin sensitivity; sulfonylureas stimulate the pancreas to release more insulin, lowering blood glucose.

Metformin Versus Sulfonylureas

Metformin had shown promise as a safer option in the blood glucose lowering biguanide group. Type 2 diabetes had formerly been known as 'maturity onset diabetes' because the condition tended to develop in persons over 40 years of age. During the 1980s, this term was replaced with 'non-insulin-dependent diabetes' with recognition of insulin resistance and the insulin-producing cells of the pancreas effectively wearing out (DeFronzo 1988; Reaven 1988).

Metformin had the ability to offset the effects of insulin resistance and resulting high glucose levels without weight gain, or glucose levels becoming too low. The benefits of metformin as a suitable treatment for non-insulin dependent type 2 diabetes gradually spread across Europe and America (Bailey and Turner 1996).

With its ability to reduce glucose formation and release by the liver, metformin was introduced in the UK by the Bristol-Myers Squibb Company in 1994. Further research showed that by increasing glucose uptake in the muscles, metformin reduced blood glucose levels by one third, and triglyceride blood fats by 10–15% (Bhattacharyya 2001). Metformin has also proved safe to be taken with sulfonylureas—which have different mechanisms and actions, the two medicines complementing one another with no contraindications (Madsen et al. 2019).

The UK Prospective Diabetes Study

In 1998, the landmark UKPDS published data on glucose-reducing treatments for 5102 patients newly diagnosed with type 2 diabetes across the UK. The study collected data from 23 diabetes clinics from 1977 to 1997 (Holman 2022). A key finding of this study showed that aside from glucose reduction, heart and circulatory system disease could be lessened by taking metformin, with clear implications for reduced severity of heart and circulatory system events (UK Prospective Diabetes Study (UKPDS) Group 1998). For patients with type 2 diabetes, where heart and blood vessel disease present a major complication risk, metformin was found to consistently and significantly reduce this risk (Holman et al. 2008).

Summary

Although sulfonylureas were initially synthesised to treat typhoid, and the effects of metformin in animal studies were discovered while searching for a malaria cure, both of these were found to reduce blood glucose levels. At last, those with type 2 diabetes had a way of controlling their condition and preventing secondary complications, triggered by consistently high blood glucose levels. Initially, metformin was not favoured as a treatment, although it eventually proved effective in reducing the amount of glucose released by the liver, and lowering the risk of cardiovascular disease in patients with type 2 diabetes. It can also be taken long-term, and does not promote weight gain, with some patients even losing weight. Today metformin is the most widely used type 2 diabetes medicine.

References

Allen F (1919) Total dietary regulations in the treatment of diabetes. Rockefeller Institute of Medical Research, New York

Bailey CJ (2017) Metformin: its botanical background. Pract Diab Int 21:115–117

Bailey CJ, Turner RC (1996) Drug therapy: metformin. N Engl J Med 334:574–579

Beckmann R (1971) Biguanide (Experimenteller Teil). Handb Exp Pharmacol 29:439–596

Bhattacharyya A (2001) Treatment of type 2 diabetes mellitus. Hosp Pharm 8:10–16

Butterfield WJ (1968) The effects of phenformin on peripheral glucose utilization and insulin action in obesity and diabetes mellitus. Ann N Y Acad Sci 148:724–733

Cavaghan MK, Ehrmann DA, Polonsky KS (2000) Interactions between insulin resistance and insulin secretion in the development of glucose intolerance. J Clin Invest 106:329–333

DeFronzo RA (1988) The triumvirate: β-cell, muscle, liver: a collusion responsible for NIDDM. Diabetes 37:667–687

Hadden DR (2005) Goat's rue—French lilac—Italian fitch—Spanish sainfoin: *Gallega officinalis* and metformin: the Edinburgh connection. J R Coll Phys Edinburgh 35:258–260

Hermann LS (1979) Metformin: a review of its pharmacological properties and therapeutic use. Diab Metab 5:233–245

Himsworth HP (1936) Diabetes mellitus: its differentiation into insulin-sensitive and insulin-insensitive types. Lancet 1:127–130

Himsworth R (2011) Sir Harold Himsworth. Diab Med 28(2):1438–1439

Holman RR (2022) A brief history of the UK prospective diabetes study. https://bjd-abcd.com/index.php/bjd/article/view/1041

Holman RR, Paul SK, Bethel AM et al (2008) 10-year follow-up of intensive glucose control in type 2 diabetes. N Engl J Med 359:1577–1589

Joslin EP (1927) The diabetic diet. J Am Diet Assoc 3:89–92

Krentz AJ, Hitman GA (2011) Sir Harold Himsworth and insulin insensitivity 75 years on. Diab Med 28(2):1435

Kroker K, Keelan J, Mazumdar PMH (2008) Crafting immunity: working histories of clinical immunology. Ashgate, Farnham, Surrey

Macleod JJR (1913) Diabetes: its pathological physiology. Arnold, London

Madsen KS, Kähler P, Kähler LK et al (2019) Metformin and second-or third-generation sulphonylurea combination therapy for adults with type 2 diabetes mellitus. Cochrane Database Syst Rev 4(4):CD012368. https://doi.org/10.1002/14651858.CD012368.pub2

Marwood SF (1973) Diabetes mellitus—some reflections. J R Coll Gen Pract 23:38–45

McKendry JB, Kuwayti K, Rado PP (1959) Clinical experience with DBI (phenformin) in the management of diabetes. Can Med Assoc J 80:773–778

Offord C (2024) Britain's post-war sugar craze confirms harms of sweet diets. Science 286(6721):475. https://pubmed.ncbi.nlm.nih.gov/39480931/

Pillans P (1998) Metformin and fatal lacticacidosis. https://www.medsafe.govt.nz/profs/puarticles/5.htm#:~:text=Lactic%20acidosis%20appears%20to%20result,those%20with%20mild%20renal%20disease

Pyke DA (1997) The history of diabetes. In: Alberti KGMM, Zimmet P, DeFronzo RA (eds) International textbook of diabetes mellitus, 2nd edn. Wiley, London

Reaven GM (1988) Role of insulin resistance in human disease. Diabetes 37:1595–1607

Schäfer G (1983) Biguanides: a review of history, pharmacodynamics and therapy. Diab Metab 9:148–163

Shapiro SL, Parrino VA, Freedman L (1959) Hypoglycemic agents III, N1-alkyl- and aralkylbiguanides. J Am Chem Soc 81:3728–3736

UK Prospective Diabetes Study (UKPDS) Group (1998) Effect of intensive blood glucose control with metformin on complications in overweight patients with type 2 diabetes (UKPDS 34). Lancet 352:854–865

7

Chronic Complications of Diabetes

In 1934, Elliot Joslin famously stated that:

> The era of the coma as the central problem of diabetes has given way to the era of complications. People with diabetes are at increased risk from the development of serious complications, including blindness, kidney failure, heart disease, stroke, and amputations. (Saunders 2002)

Following the discovery of insulin, diabetic comas due to high blood glucose levels were reduced from over 60% to 5% (Joslin 1934). However, there was no established limit regarding how much glucose the human body could tolerate. It was clear that high glucose levels increased to risk of long-term complications, but before the introduction of insulin many people with diabetes did not live long enough to develop these secondary health problems. Today in the UK, nearly 6% of the National Health budget is spent on treating largely preventable complications of diabetes (University of York 2024).

Most complications of diabetes are the result of poor blood supply, which damages nerves, blood vessels and organs. A continually high blood glucose level means the heart has to work much harder as the blood is thicker, and consequently smaller blood vessels become blocked, causing death of the tissue beyond this point. Chronic complications can develop *after* 10 years of previous poor control, even if glucose control has been good for several years following this period (Shaw and Cummings 2005).

Some people are more susceptible to chronic complications, due to factors such as ethnicity, genetic factors, duration of diabetes and age. Elevated

V. Wilson, *Diabetes Ancient and Modern*, Hippocrates,
https://doi.org/10.1007/978-3-032-12454-8_7

glucose levels can also lead to the release of a protein, kinase-C, resulting in the unnatural division of body cells, and the possibility of developing cancers (Barnett and Grice 2011).

Advancing Knowledge of Complications

A long-term study reported in 1978 showed that small blood vessel disease is one of the first chronic complications to develop in both type 1 and type 2 diabetes (Tchobroutsky 1978). Studies have also shown that high glucose levels over time cause nerve (neurological) damage, as well as heart and major blood vessel disease (macrovascular complications).

Fact

A groundbreaking study showed that over ten years, good control of blood glucose levels reduces the development of kidney disease (nephropathy) in diabetes by 34%, and later stage kidney disease by 56%. In addition, nerve disease (neuropathy), and eye disease (retinopathy) risk were also significantly reduced (Diabetes Control and Complications Trial (DCCT) 1993).

A second study in 1995 showed that controlling glucose levels significantly reduced heart and blood vessel disease, although research participants were below 40 years of age, possibly a factor impacting the results (DCCT 1995).

Similarly, the 1998 UKPDS study showed that good control of glucose levels in type 2 diabetes resulted in a 21% reduced rate of retinopathy, and a 29% reduction in patients requiring laser eye treatment (UK Prospective Diabetes Study (UKPDS) 1998); a reduction in the development of kidney disease, and a 16% fall in heart disease (Fowler 2008).

It is now known that glucose attaches to red blood cells; the amount of glucose present over the three-month life of the red blood cell is measured in an HbA1c test (glycosylated haemoglobin test). The normal range for glucose in the blood is 4–7 mmol/L (72–126 mg/dL measurement in the U.S.). The closer blood glucose levels are to normal (around 6%), the lower the risk of developing complications. It is possible for glucose to attach to white blood cells, and if levels are too high, this can change how the white cells work to fight infection, and alter how red blood cells take up oxygen.

Large amounts of glucose within the blood changes the way the glucose can be used by the body. Complications can also be triggered in this way, as glucose is broken down into sorbitol as energy is produced. High levels of sorbitol can alter fluid balance. Sorbitol becomes trapped, causing damage to the cellular structure if the fluid balance is equal both inside and outside the cell (Barnett and Grice 2011).

The cost of treating complications increases each year due to the number of people developing diabetes.

With the availability of fast food in the Western world, rates of obesity and related type 2 diabetes are escalating, and consequently treatment costs for diabetes and its complications are also rapidly rising. In many, if not most cases, type 2 diabetes is triggered by a high-calorie, high-fat diet, with little or no exercise.

Historical Observations on Complications

Before the advent of insulin, people with diabetes tended to die before chronic complications could develop, and any additional health problems were not attributed to diabetes as they would be now. Due to limited life expectancy, there are few historical reports of complications in people with diabetes.

Cataract surgery has been performed since ancient times, as has treatment for leg ulcers, although not specifically recognised as a direct consequence of diabetes. Because they were uncommon, and due to lack of recognition regarding the cause, the complications of diabetes were rarely mentioned in historical accounts. Tingling in the feet and legs, or veiled vision, which would be recognised today as complications of diabetes, would not have been seen as a secondary condition associated with the primary diabetes.

Historical Observations on Diabetic Nerve Disease (Neuropathy)

It was not until the nineteenth century that a causal link between diabetes and nervous system disease was finally made.

What Is Neuropathy?

Neuropathy (nerve damage) can occur in any part of the body due to long-term high blood glucose levels. Neuropathy is now categorised into several different types:

- Peripheral neuropathy affects the nerves in the hands and feet (extremities).
- Diffuse neuropathies appear as altered sensations in the hands and feet.
- Distal polyneuropathy results in a reduced ability to detect pain and temperature, with tingling, burning, severe nerve pain, sensitivity to touch, and loss of balance or coordination. This condition worsens with duration of both type 1 and type 2 diabetes, affecting as many as 60% of patients; neuropathy increases the risk of developing diabetic eye and kidney disease (Tesfaye and Boulton 2009).

In the ancient Orient, there was recognition of nerve pain in the lower limbs of patients with diabetes in the eighth century. The first modern association between diabetes and peripheral neuropathy was made in 1864 by *Marchal de Calvi*, a French doctor.

A further advance came after two decades when *Althaus*, a German physician added to existing knowledge regarding symptoms, such as foot pain that became more severe at night than during the day (Althaus 1884).

Also in 1884, *Bouchard* made the association between patients having no knee-jerk reaction due to severe nerve damage in the lower limbs (Bouchard 1884).

In 1885, *Pavy*, a Victorian diabetes specialist from London, noted from his numerous diabetic patients a link between high glucose levels in the blood and multiple occurrences of peripheral neuropathy. He described (Pavy 1885):

> Heavy legs, numb feet, lightening pain and deep-seated pain in the feet, hyperaesthesia [extreme sensitivity to touch], muscle tenderness, and impairment of patellar [knee] tendon reflexes.

The nerve pain was such that Pavy could only offer his patients opium, as diabetes treatments at this time had no ability to significantly reverse high blood glucose levels.

In 1887, *Davies Pryce*, a Nottingham surgeon, noted the inflammation and structural changes in the nerves of the hands and feet, also observing the association between slow-healing foot ulcers due to poor blood supply (Pryce 1887):

> It will be seen that a good many of the causes which have been believed to produce perforating ulcers were also present—cold, alcohol, diabetes, vascular disease and continued pressure. It is probable that all these played a part in the causation of disease but I would venture to assign a considerable share to diabetes and vascular disease.

Even today, the first sign of type 2 diabetes may be a non-healing foot ulcer. Other than accidents, poor blood supply to the lower limbs is the most common reason for amputation, with lower limb amputation being 15–40 times more likely in patients with diabetes (Fowler 2008).

Pryce's observations provided insight into the reasons why foot ulcers develop in diabetes, including that the shape of the foot changes to increase pressure in certain areas so an ulcer develops, and also peripheral neuropathy and the impact of reduced blood supply.

In 1887, a further advance in the understanding of peripheral neuropathy came when *Layden*, a German physician, categorised each of the symptomatic changes that occur in peripheral nerve damage (Layden 1887):

Stage 1: Excessive sensitivity to touch or neuralgic (nerve pain) form
Stage 2: Motor or paralytic form, referring to the type of nerve damage
Stage 3: Absence of co-ordination and muscle function with altered or staggering gait

Purdy, another nineteenth-century doctor with an interest in nerve damage, stated: 'It is rare to meet with a case of diabetes in which there is not more or less nervous disturbance' (Purdy 1890).

Nerve damage can also cause arthritic changes in the feet, reduced sensation and pressure build-up. This degenerative condition of the foot was named 'Charcot joints' after the French neurologist *Jean-Matin Charcot* in 1890. Charcot observed that diabetic patients with peripheral nerve damage in the feet walked with an altered gait and increasingly poor co-ordination. He took photos to document these conditions and went on to describe the medical abnormalities of Charcot disease (Charcot 1890). He stated that patients commonly:

> complain about flashing pain existing for 18 months which wakes him up at night. The pain occurs five or six times a day, followed by hyperaesthesia [extreme sensitivity to touch]. He also has pins and needles in his legs which prevent him from feeling the nature of the floor. He always feels too hot or too cold in his feet; on physical examination he is completely absent of patellar reflexes.

What Is Autonomic Neuropathy?

Autonomic neuropathy concerns damage to the autonomic nerves that control the unconscious functions that we don't have to think about, such as breathing, heartbeat and digestive function. This type of neuropathy is significant and unfortunately common, again due to long-term high blood glucose levels. These various autonomic complications may go unrecognised or, in the case of digestive issues in diabetes, be mistaken for irritable bowel syndrome when it is in fact delayed stomach emptying due to nerve damage (Vinik et al. 2003).

Autonomic neuropathy can exist alongside peripheral nerve damage or be present on its own. A variety of studies have demonstrated that the number of patients developing autonomic nerve damage ranges from 16.8% to 50%, and that with good control of glucose levels, these conditions can become stable (Tesfaye and Boulton 2009).

In 1798, *John Rollo* explained the consequences of nerve damage to stomach function, describing one of his patients as (Rollo 1798):

> His skin is dry, his face flushed. He is frequently sick and throws up matter of a viscid nature, and of bitterish, and sweetish taste. After eating he has a pain of his stomach, which continues for half an hour… [Rollo goes on to describe additional damage to the genito-urinary system nerves] He makes much urine, 10–12 pints in the 24 hours, to the voiding of which he has urgent propensities peculiarly distressing to him, and constantly dribbling.

Rollo did not draw a connection between these symptoms and diabetic nerve damage. His documented evidence describes the condition we know today as gastroparesis—slow emptying of the stomach, bloating and diarrhoea or constipation.

Historical Observations on Kidney Disease

Historical Observations on Diabetic Kidney Disease (Nephropathy)

Throughout history, diabetes has always been thought of as a disease of the kidneys due to the symptoms of great thirst (known medically as polydipsia) and frequently passing large quantities of urine (polyuria).

Diabetic kidney disease describes a continuous and detectable amount of protein in the urine, linked with high blood pressure and reduced kidney function. Today we know that diabetic nephropathy has varying stages of severity. This very common complication of diabetes is the leading cause of chronic kidney disease and end-stage renal (kidney) disease (ESRD) in developed countries, including the United States (Rout and Jialal 2025).

The link between diabetes and reduced renal function was first observed in the eighteenth century by the physician *Cotunnius*, who reported the presence of protein in the urine (proteinuria) in diabetes in 1764 (Williamson 1840). Seventy-two years later in 1836, *Bright* found that albumin—a protein—in the urine was linked to kidney disease, although the reason for this was not understood. Similarly, this observation of diabetic kidney disease was also made by *Pierre Rayer* (1793–1867) (Rayner et al. 2005).

Bernard Naunyn later observed that 'a small amount of albumin (protein) in the urine of a patient with diabetes was not a concern, but a large amount should be seen as a bad prognostic sign' (Lee 2000). We now know that a small amount of protein is known as micro-albuminuria, while a large amount is an indication that the kidneys are failing.

American physician *William Osler* (1849–1919) wrote *The Principles and Practice of Medicine*, in which he states that protein in the urine in diabetic patients is (Osler 1982):

> A tolerably frequent complication. The amount varies greatly and, when slight, does not seem to be of much moment. It is associated with atherosclerosis [narrowing of the arteries due to fatty deposits]. It occasionally precedes the development of diabetic coma.

In 1934, hardening of the kidneys and tissue damage was first noted by *Elliot Joslin* in association with high glucose levels, a major cause of all complications of diabetes (Shiskin 1950). Even today, diabetes is the leading cause of end-stage kidney disease in the Western world (Diabetes UK 2023). It has also been recognised that diabetic kidney disease is associated with increased risk for cardiovascular complications (Diabetes UK 2023).

Complications: What We Now Know

There is not a single part of the human body that remains unaffected by diabetes. As blood flow is essential for every part of the body to survive, any abnormality has the potential to cause disease. Diabetes affects the body at a cellular level, and the discovery of insulin has not prevented the onset of complications, which occur due to factors such as how well blood glucose levels are managed, duration of diabetes, genetics, ethnicity, age and environment.

Insulin has slowed the onset and reduced the severity of chronic complications of diabetes. Complications appear in many cases to be inevitable over time, due to metabolic changes, raising the question of whether complications will occur anyway, no matter how good the control (Rask-Madsen and King 2013). Metabolic function within the cells cannot be normal in diabetes: there is no such thing as perfect control of blood glucose levels. However, it is important to manage blood glucose as well as possible to within the normal range to reduce the rate of progression and increase life expectancy.

Undiagnosed diabetes is a major concern, potentially leading to serious complications due to unrecognised high blood glucose levels. Early diagnosis is essential to lessen and delay chronic complications, although it is possible for type 2 diabetes to remain undiagnosed for many years because the symptoms are slow to develop (Diabetes UK 2025).

In the UK, it is estimated that 1 million people are currently living with undiagnosed type 2 diabetes, meaning that around one third of people living with type 2 are unaware they have it. Prediabetes, where blood glucose levels are higher than normal but not high enough for a diabetes diagnosis, affects around 5.1 million adults in England (Office for National Statistics 2019).

Lifestyle factors, such as smoking, make complications more likely to develop. Both smoking and diabetes independently increase the risk of cardiovascular complications, such as heart attack, stroke and circulatory system disease, with smoking making this risk much higher in people with diabetes. Smoking can also worsen diabetic eye, nerve and kidney disease (United States Food and Drug Administration 2024).

Mental Wellbeing

Unsurprisingly, diabetes self-management is very demanding as the patient carries out 95% of their self-care activities, such as glucose monitoring, insulin and medicine administration, dietary management and taking regular exercise. Emotional distress and mental health problems are common in association with a poorer quality of life with diabetic complications, and increased physical impairment.

Patients may not follow the guidance of healthcare professionals, although this may be due to reasoned decision-making (Vahdat et al. 2014); for example a patient may not take prescribed pain medicine if they have constipation, as strong painkillers make diabetic constipation worse. Although informed choice is a principle of patient empowerment, the patient may be unable to carry out medical instructions; for example a patient who has diabetes and severe depression may find it difficult to adhere to their diabetes and depression treatment regimes.

Patients with diabetes often choose to undertake some but not all expected self-care behaviours. This may be based on personal or religious health beliefs, or purely because the patient does not want to or chooses not to follow a complex medical regime (Wilson 2022).

Depression and diabetes go together, although they are both separate health conditions: diabetes often results in depression, and a period of depression can trigger type 2 diabetes. Varying factors trigger a state of depression, although this may go undiagnosed despite the association between depression and a reduction in diabetes self-care activities. Depression is three times more common in those with diabetes than in the general population (Kalton et al. 2010).

Patients with diabetes often experience severe and recurrent depression throughout their lives, with research indicating that females with diabetes are more likely to have depression than males, with depression occurring at similar rates in type 1 and type 2 diabetes (Clark 2003).

Various factors are associated with depression in diabetes, including poor glucose control, a long duration of diabetes and the development and level of impairment of complications such as sight difficulties (Park et al. 2013).

It is necessary for patients with diabetes to have their HbA1c tested every 3–6 months, as well as cholesterol and blood pressure monitoring, and to receive annual eye screening for retinopathy, renal function screening and foot checks to detect any changes at the earliest possible stage.

Summary

High blood glucose levels in diabetes can potentially lead to a number of different complications, such as blindness, heart and circulatory disease, impaired kidney function and nerve damage. Before the discovery of insulin patients had their lives limited by diabetes, and few lived long enough to develop chronic complications. With the use of insulin, patients lived longer but developed complications because blood glucose levels were not kept within normal range.

We now know that chronic complications can be delayed and stabilised with good glucose control to reduce the amount of glucose sticking to red blood cells (tested as HbA1c). However, the Diabetes Control and Complications Trial (1993) could not define the specific level at which delay or stabilisation would be effective. A target of around <7.0% (53 mmol/mol) is typically recommended for most adults with diabetes to prevent long-term complications.

A stricter target of <6.5% (48 mmol/mol) may be appropriate for selected patients who are younger, in good health, have a short duration of diabetes, a long life expectancy, and are not at high risk of hypoglycaemia (low blood sugar).

A less stringent or relaxed target, often in the range of 7.5% to 8.0% or higher, is generally recommended for patients who are older, have a history of severe hypoglycaemia, limited life expectancy, extensive co-morbidities, or established chronic complications (such as heart or kidney disease). In these cases, the risks associated with intensive glucose-lowering therapy (primarily hypoglycaemia) often outweigh the potential long-term benefits.

Diabetes is predominantly self-managed by the individual with the condition, meaning that the risk of not actively controlling blood glucose levels must be properly understood to be aware of the consequences. Psycho-social factors presenting barriers to good control of diabetes were previously not widely understood. We now know glucose control is affected by lifestyle factors such as stress, emotional upset or illness, depression and diabetes medicines. The individual's own attitude towards, and the ability to carry out, necessary diabetes self-management activities is therefore vitally important.

References

Althaus J (1884) Ueber Sklerose des Rückenmarkes. Otto Wigand, Leipzig

Barnett AH, Grice J (2011) New mechanisms in glucose control. Wiley, Chichester

Bouchard C (1884) Sur la perte des reflexes tendineux dans la diabètes sucré. Progrés Médicine 12:819

Charcot JM (1890) Sur un casa de paraplegic diabetique. Reprinted in Ward JD. In: Boulton AJMT (ed) Historical aspects of diabetic peripheral neuropathy. Bridgewater, Aventis

Clark M (2003) Identification and treatment of depression in people with diabetes. Diabetes Primary Care 5(3):124–127

Diabetes UK (2023) Diabetes and heart disease. www.diabetes.org.uk/guide-t0-diabetes/complications/cardiovascular_disease

Diabetes UK (2025) Diabetes risk factors. https://www.diabetes.org.uk/about-diabetes/type-2-diabetes/diabetes-risk-factors

Fowler MJ (2008) Microvascular and macrovascular complications of diabetes. Clin Diabetes 26(2):77–82

Joslin E. (1934) The menace of diabetic gangrene. New Eng J Med 211: 19–20. https://www.nejm.org/doi/full/10.1056/nejm193407052110103

Kalton W, Maj M, Sartorius N (2010) Depression and diabetes. Wiley-Blackwell, Chichester

Layden R (1887) Die entzundung der peripheren nerven. Deut Militar Zaitsch 17:49

Lee HSJ (2000) Dates in urology: a chronological record in urology over the last millennium. Informative Health-care, California

Office for National Statistics (2019) Risk factors for pre-diabetes and undiagnosed type 2 diabetes in England: 2013 to 2019. https://www.ons.gov.uk/peoplepopulationandcommunity/healthandsocialcare/healthinequalities/bulletins/riskfactorsforprediabetesandundiagnosedtype2diabetesinengland/2013to2019#:~:text=1.,to%20approximately%205.1%20million%20adults

Osler W (1982) The principles and practice of medicine. Classics of Medicine Library, Birmingham

Park M, Kalton WJ, Wolf FM et al (2013) Depression and risk of mortality in individuals with diabetes: a meta-analysis and systematic review. Gen Hosp Psychiatry 35(3):217–225

Pavy FW (1885) Introductory address to the discussion on the clinical aspects of glycosuria. Lancet 2:1085–1087

Pryce TD (1887) Perforating ulcers of both feet associated with diabetes and ataxic symptoms. Lancet 2:11–12

Purdy, C.W. (1890) Diabetes—its causes, symptoms and treatment. Great Malvern: Book on Demand Publishing

Rask-Madsen, C., and King, G.L. (2013) Vascular complications of diabetes: mechanisms of injury and protective factors. Cell Metab 8; 17(1): 20–33

Rayner P-FO, Berry D, Mackenzie D et al (2005) The history of albuminous nephritis (1940). The Wellcome Trust Centre for the History of Medicine at University College London, London

Rollo J (1798) Cases of the diabetes mellitus with the results of the trials of certain acids. T. Gilles for C. Dilly, C, London

Rout P, Jialal I (2025) Diabetic nephropathy. https://www.ncbi.nlm.nih.gov/books/NBK534200/

Saunders I (2002) From Thebes to Toronto and the 21st century: an incredible journey. Diab Spectr 15:56–60

Shaw, K.M. and Cummings, M.H. (2005) Diabetes: chronic complications. 2nd, Chichester: Wiley

Shiskin C (1950) Correspondence. Br Med J 1490

Tchobroutsky G (1978) Relation of diabetic control to development of microvascular complications. Diabetologia 15(3):143–152

Tesfaye S, Boulton A (2009) Diabetic neuropathy. Oxford University Press, Oxford

The Diabetes Control and Complications Trial (DCCT) Research Group (1993) The effect of intensive treatment of diabetes on the development and treatment and progression of long-term complications in insulin-dependent diabetes mellitus. N Engl J Med 329:977–034

The Diabetes Control and Complications Trial (DCCT) Research Group (1995) Effect of intensive diabetes management on the macrovascular events and risk factors in the Diabetes Control and Complications Trial. Am J Cardiol 75:894–903

The UK Prospective Diabetes Study (UKPDS) Group (1998) Effect of intensive blood glucose control with sulfonylureas or insulin compared with conventional treatment and risk of complications in patients with type 2 diabetes (UKPDS 33). Lancet 352:837–853

United States Food and Drug Administration (2024) How smoking can increase risk and affect diabetes. https://www.fda.gov/tobacco-products/health-effects-tobacco-use/how-smoking-can-increase-risk-and-affect-diabetes

University of York (2024) Cost of diabetes to UK estimated at £14 billion, research shows. https://www.york.ac.uk/news-and-events/news/2024/research/diabetes-cost-to-uk/

Vahdat S, Hemzehgardeshi L, Hessam S, et al (2014) Patient involvement in health-care decision-making: a review. https://pmc.ncbi.nlm.nih.gov/articles/PMC3964421/

Vinik AI, Maser RE, Mitchell BD et al (2003) Diabetic autonomic neuropathy. Diabetes Care 25(3):1553

Williamson T (1840) Edinburgh medical and surgical journal: exhibiting a concise view of the latest and most important discoveries in medicine, surgery and pharmacy, Edinburgh

Wilson V (2022) Psychology in diabetes care and practice. Routledge, Abingdon

8

Further Advances

Diabetes is a disease that must be self-managed, where the individual is responsible for day-to-day control of their condition; patients with diabetes are responsible for 99% of their self-care. Although specialised technology is available in many countries, it is not in all, and the individual still has to be willing to use the technology correctly so it assists in monitoring blood glucose levels.

As we have seen in previous chapters, the causal link between consistently high glucose levels and chronic complications has now been firmly established. The level of glycaemic (blood glucose) control can be seen in an HbA1c test that shows the amount of glucose sticking to the red blood cells over the previous 3 months. However, an HbA1c result gives an average of highs and lows. This means that control could be poor on one day, with high glucose levels, and within or lower than normal range on another which does not equate to good control. Unfortunately, the HbA1c remains the standard test of blood glucose control in many countries.

In recent years, psychosocial issues have been recognised as a major influence on diabetes self-care. There is now a clear link that was not previously understood between high blood glucose levels and rates of depression, anxiety, stress, illness and other lifestyle factors. These external factors increase blood glucose levels due to hormonal interactions, and it may be very difficult for diabetes control to be achieved. Depression may also lead to type 2 diabetes by increasing blood glucose levels over time.

Depression can be caused by diabetes and equally, diabetes can be caused by depression.

V. Wilson, *Diabetes Ancient and Modern*, Hippocrates,
https://doi.org/10.1007/978-3-032-12454-8_8

The DAFNE Diabetes Education Course

The Dosage Adjustment for Normal Eating (DAFNE) education course for adults with type 1 diabetes was designed in 2000. The five-day structured course focuses on working out carbohydrate values and learning to give an appropriate insulin dose for this amount of carbohydrate. This course is delivered by trained health educators and helps the individual to self-manage their diabetes and lifestyle day-to-day. The programme also teaches peak insulin action times to avoid and manage low glucose levels, monitoring blood glucose levels and managing glucose levels during illness, after drinking alcohol and when exercising.

The Advent of Diabetes Technology

Technology—predominantly to assist management of type 1 diabetes—has sought to provide ways to attain normalised blood glucose levels.

Continuous Subcutaneous Insulin Infusion (CSII)

CSII, or insulin pump therapy, can be traced back to the late 1970s. The idea was to introduce insulin directly under the skin in controlled continuous small doses to closely mimic the body's normal insulin release (Fredrickson 1995). This groundbreaking piece of technology was originally the size of a rucksack, but as medical device research has advanced, modern insulin pumps are now the size of a small mobile phone.

An insulin pump consists of a reservoir containing insulin within a syringe, connected to tubing which leads to a small plastic cannula (hollow tube) which is inserted via a needle under the skin. This stays in place to deliver continuous insulin for 2–3 days before the site is changed; infusion can be into the abdomen, arms or thighs (Wilson 2003). The insulin pump user learns to change the tubing and fill the insulin reservoir, having received patient education from their diabetes team.

It must be noted that changing the infusion set halts insulin flow, potentially resulting in temporarily raised blood glucose levels. There can then follow a sharp decrease in blood glucose levels a few hours later due to insulin pooling around the infusion site (Wilson 2003). It is therefore vitally important for blood glucose levels to be regularly tested by the patient.

An insulin pump can be programmed so that the rate of insulin delivery may be increased or decreased according to need. Blood glucose levels should be tested regularly (4–6 times a day), especially during illness, before bed or driving a vehicle (Wilson 2005). Insulin pumps have now advanced to such a degree that a built-in glucose sensor measures plasma glucose and delivers insulin automatically as an 'artificial pancreas'.

Insulin pump therapy is an alternative to multiple daily injections (MDI), providing improved blood glucose control, and reducing episodes of low blood glucose when compared with injections (Pickup 2009). Advantages of insulin pump therapy include:

- Delaying the onset of chronic complications (DCCT Research Group 1993, 1996).
- Improved blood glucose levels during pregnancy (Gabbe et al. 2000; Skyler 2000).
- An overall achievement in controlling blood glucose levels to lead a normal lifestyle, such as eating at unscheduled times, or having a restaurant meal (Walsh and Roberts 1999).

Following the initial cost of an insulin pump and ongoing consumables, this cost to the National Health Service (NHS) is outweighed considerably by the prevention of chronic complications and the cost of treating them. In the UK alone, chronic complications account for one in five coronary (heart) hospital admissions (The National Diabetes Support Team 2005). Instrumental in achieving funding for patients needing pump therapy in the UK, the author carried out necessary research to show the Department of Health that insulin pump therapy could prevent complications, save money and improve quality of life (Wilson and Davis 2004).

Continuous Glucose Monitoring

Blood glucose meter readings are a snapshot in time and do not show overall trends of good or poor control. A continuous glucose monitoring (CGM) system, as the name suggests, takes continual glucose readings, depicting all the fluctuations throughout the day and night. The advantage is that this system allows the user to know their glucose levels and trends, so that insulin dosage can be altered accordingly. This is a huge advance in the prevention of complications.

The CGM works in conjunction with an insulin pump to manage diabetes effectively. It is therefore vitally important that thorough training is given to the patient (Pickup 2009; Burgess et al. 2008). CGM sensors are placed under the skin and read plasma glucose levels every 5 min, sending a signal to the insulin pump. This data, shown in graph form, can be downloaded by the patient's diabetes specialist. The sensors continue to work for roughly 6 days, requiring finger-prick blood glucose monitoring to ensure proper calibration and accurate readings.

In the same way, flash glucose monitoring sensors are currently used by patients with type 1 or type 2 diabetes. The sensor is placed beneath the skin in the same way, although it does not give continual plasma glucose readings, requiring the patient to swipe their smartphone over the sensor to send a reading to the phone to see their glucose level. However, the FreeStyle Libre glucose sensor can be used with a compatible smartphone to provide real-time continuous glucose readings.

Plasma glucose levels are not the same as blood glucose levels, and the difference can be as much as 2 mmol/L higher or lower than blood glucose readings. This shows that it is still important to regularly test blood glucose levels, especially before basing an insulin dose on these readings, or driving a vehicle. The use of CGM is especially beneficial for patients who no longer have warning signs of low glucose levels so that action can be taken quickly (Klondoff et al. 2011; Bergenstal et al. 2010; Pickup 2009).

Modern blood testing strips directly monitor plasma, rather than whole blood. This may be problematic for patients with type 1 diabetes who have frequent and unpredictable low glucose levels as the difference between 5 mmol/L plasma glucose and 3 mmol/L whole blood is significant—the difference between a normal blood glucose level and a low level, requiring action to treat hypoglycaemia (the medical term for low blood glucose). Hypoglycaemia is defined as a blood glucose level below 4 mmol/L (72 mg/dL).

Transplantation

Before the discovery of insulin, attempts at pancreatic transplantation were made. In 1894, Patrick Watson-Williams implanted a sheep's pancreas under the skin of a 15-year-old boy with type 1 diabetes. The surgery failed to cure the patient due to a lack of understanding of compatibility and how the islet cells work, and the boy died a few days later (Tattersall 1995). Although pancreatic transplant surgery was available as early as 1966, it became more feasible in 1978 (Sutherland and Gruessner 1997). However, success rates were low. This was mainly due to the use of immunosuppressant drugs to prevent rejection, which were destroying the new insulin-producing cells in the transplanted pancreas (Robertson et al. 1998).

Since the year 2000, the survival rate of patients who have received a transplanted pancreas has risen to 95%, although some physicians feel this type of surgery is controversial (Sutherland and Gruessner 2001).

Patients with type 1 diabetes who have significant kidney impairment could be candidates for a joint kidney and pancreatic transplant (Wass et al. 2011; Kaufman and Sutherland 2011). This 'graft' procedure has been shown to significantly improve the patient's quality of life, enabling attainment of normal HbA1c levels. This surgery is not commonly performed as the patient must meet certain criteria, such as very unstable blood glucose levels, recurrent episodes of ketoacidosis and poor effectiveness of insulin (Hakim et al. 2010; Knoll and Nichol 2003).

Patients undergoing this surgery have worse health outcomes in comparison with patients who take multiple daily insulin injections (Venstrom et al. 2003). It is unusual for patients with type 2 diabetes to be considered for a joint kidney and pancreas transplant procedure; the majority of surgery is performed on patients with type 1 diabetes, with only 10% of transplants being for patients with type 2 (Sampaio et al. 2011). Success rates are equal to those in type 1 diabetes (Knoll and Nichol 2003). Due to surgical complications a combined kidney and pancreas transplant has high risks compared with the kidney or pancreatic procedure alone, for reasons such as infection, rejection and the need for anti-rejection drugs (Hakim et al. 2010; Wass et al. 2011).

Transplantation of Pancreatic Islet Cells

In the 1990s, injected treatment of insulin-producing cells was undertaken to restore normal insulin function (Wass et al. 2011). This procedure was seen to be less invasive than a full pancreatic transplant; however, this required more than 300,000 islet cells to be harvested, although this has been shown to successfully reverse type 1 diabetes over time (Ryan et al. 2005). Better understanding of the embryonic pancreas has led to increased knowledge in this area (Wang et al. 2012).

Due to the quantity of islet cells required, there is a problem with availability of deceased donors (living pancreas transplants are not performed in the UK), reducing the number of procedures that can be undertaken, and animal trials continue. Transplanting organs from animal donors to humans is called *xenotransplantation*. Genetically modified pigs bred specially for this process to lower the risk of rejection is a promising development. Current research is looking at ways to protect human islet cells from destruction by the body's immune system (Fang et al. 2024).

The Potential of Embryonic Cells

There are two main types of body cells that could potentially produce insulin: embryonic and adult. Embryonic cells can be turned into any other cell in the body for a limited period (Totey and Deb 2010). However, over-manipulated embryonic cells can suffer from overgrowth which can lead to tumours (Efrats 2009). Adult stem cells can be sourced from bone marrow and chemically manipulated to create more. Unfortunately, adult stem cells are affected by impurity issues that create difficulty in changing them into insulin-producing beta islet cells (Khan 2011).

It has been proven under laboratory conditions that a single islet cell in isolation does not work as well as a cluster of cells (Efrats 2009). Consequently, the lower the number of cells, the less insulin that is produced (Khan 2011).

Developments in stem cell technology using the patient's own bone marrow is ongoing, specifically stem cell transplants, where a patient's own stem cells are collected and later returned after treatment. This method is used to treat various conditions like certain cancers. Research carried out in Brazil in 2008 showed that 20 out of 23 patients reported that they no longer needed insulin injections following a stem cell transplant to produce islet cells, with an average HbA1c within normal range (Couri and Volterelli 2009).

Further advances in this treatment technology are looking at stem cells derived from islet cell transplants for type 1 diabetes; this research is currently being conducted in Oxford, UK (Diabetes Research and Wellness Foundation 2023). This procedure requires a huge number of islet cells for implantation, and the patient must remain on anti-rejection drugs to prevent the body from destroying these implanted islets cells.

An alternative field of research is to isolate the autoimmune destructive factor in type 1 diabetes that continually destroys the insulin-producing cells. It is now possible to create embryonic stem cells that are immune to this attack (Hakim et al. 2010). Clinical trials using adult stem cells from the patient have successfully managed to treat heart disease. Using the patient's own stem cells has the advantage of reducing the chances of rejection and the use of anti-rejection drugs.

In some countries, embryonic stem cell research is a controversial topic based on religious beliefs and moral grounds. It is important in all aspects of medicine that scientific research can continue. We can see throughout history that without scientific and medical advance, tens of millions of people would not be alive today.

Reversing Prediabetes and Type 2 Diabetes

Patients with type 2 diabetes are often able to improve their blood glucose control with weight loss and regular exercise to allow insulin to work more efficiently. However, factors such as age, ethnicity, genetics and duration of diabetes mean that the condition cannot be completely reversed, and if weight is regained, type 2 diabetes returns.

The World Health Organisation has estimated that up to 90% of people who go on to develop type 2 diabetes are classified as obese (WHO 2011).

In the presence of excess body fat, cells cannot use insulin effectively to reduce blood glucose levels and use or store this glucose for fuel. Type 2 diabetes often develops very slowly, with the body gradually becoming less able to regulate glucose levels. It may take many years before symptoms such as increased thirst and slow healing are recognised as due to prediabetes or type 2 diabetes, and a diagnosis may not be made until after chronic complications have developed (Diabetes UK 2008).

Healthcare providers are seeing the escalating cost of treating type 2 diabetes and complications, especially with medicines to help the body make more insulin and to improve insulin sensitivity as new diagnoses are made. With diet, regular exercise and weight loss it is possible to reverse prediabetes and type 2 diabetes in many cases. By making these changes to lifestyle, blood glucose levels are reduced because the body can use insulin more efficiently.

Research has shown that by losing 5–7% of bodyweight, the risk of type 2 diabetes developing is reduced considerably, and pre-existing type 2 or prediabetes can be improved or reversed with blood glucose levels within normal range (Diabetes UK 2025).

Problems with maintaining a healthy weight typically start around the teenage years, where factors such as anxiety and depression, a sedentary lifestyle and irregular eating patterns begin, which then establish future adult eating and exercise behaviour (Wilson 2022).

Some people cannot reverse their type 2 diabetes. If blood glucose levels are high due to factors such as genetics, age, ethnicity, other medical conditions or as a consequence of necessary medications, these are risk factors that cannot be altered. However, weight loss and increased exercise will still improve blood glucose levels and overall health. The following dietary and exercise changes are advised for improvement or reversal of prediabetes and type 2 diabetes.

The DESMOND Type 2 Diabetes Education Course

The Diabetes Education and Self-Management for Ongoing and Newly Diagnosed (DESMOND) course was designed in 2006 to help individuals with type 2 diabetes better understand and manage their condition. This programme of structured group education aims to improve knowledge about diabetes to promote healthy lifestyle choices, giving patients the confidence to better self-manage their type 2 diabetes. The course is usually run by trained or lay healthcare educators in community venues or primary care settings.

Lifestyle Changes

Eating a healthy diet to improve or beat prediabetes and type 2 diabetes involves awareness of food choices. Highly processed foods (refined carbohydrates) like white bread, most breakfast cereals, white rice, biscuits, cakes, pastry, crisps and fast food should be avoided, as they are high in sugar, fat and salt. A healthy choice is whole foods that have not been processed, including vegetables, fruits (not high-sugar pineapple or mango), brown rice, wholegrain bread and pulses, such as chickpeas and lentils. Drinks containing a high level of sugar are not a healthy choice, and even though fruit smoothies look healthy because they contain fruit, they contain high levels of fruit sugar (fructose), which raises cholesterol if consumed in excess.

Unhealthy, saturated animal fats, such as butter, lard and ghee, should be replaced by fats such as rapeseed oil, which is lower in calories than olive oil. Palm oil is especially bad for increasing cholesterol; palm oil is high in saturated fats and is an ingredient in many foods. It is important to read food labels to assess the levels of sugar, fat and salt; if sugar is the first, second or third ingredient, then that product is high in sugar.

Blood glucose levels can be regulated by dietary fibre. In the UK it is recommended that 30g of dietary fibre should be eaten daily. This slows the absorption of glucose in the intestines, lowering blood glucose levels, and reducing the risk of prediabetes and type 2 diabetes. A healthy intake of dietary fibre is energy-rich and filling, promoting weight loss; fibre has a beneficial effect on the absorption of dietary fats and cholesterol, and helps reduce inflammation and blood pressure.

Movement

Any movement counts as exercise, and this does not have to be done at a gym; a small amount of physical effort has real health benefits. It is recommended that for a healthy lifestyle, 150 minutes of exercise is taken each week. This can be divided into smaller sessions that add up to a total of 150 minutes, involving activities like walking the dog every day, walking the children to school or climbing stairs. The aim is to do an activity regularly that gets you slightly out of breath.

Moving more has a number of health benefits. Regular physical activity helps the body use insulin more effectively by increasing the sensitivity of body cells to insulin, preventing unused glucose from accumulating in the blood. Additionally, exercise can help to reduce weight gain, which is a significant factor in the development of prediabetes and type 2 diabetes.

Other Lifestyle Factors

Sleep is important to glucose metabolism, and constantly waking up, or too little sleep increases blood glucose levels. Research has convincingly shown that getting less than 6 hours of sleep each night increases fasting blood glucose levels. This makes prediabetes and type 2 diabetes 4.5 times more likely (Darraj 2023).

Smoking is a habit that does not go well with diabetes. People who smoke are 30–40% more likely to develop type 2 diabetes than those who don't smoke (Centre for Disease Control 2004). Nicotine thickens the blood, making the heart work harder. This increases the risk of heart disease, stroke and circulatory complications already associated with type 2 diabetes.

Metabolic syndrome describes a group of associated conditions or risk factors that accompany type 2 diabetes, including obesity, coronary heart disease, high blood pressure, high blood fats such as cholesterol and chemicals that prevent blood clots in the arteries and heart from breaking down. Prediabetes, due to excess body fat and an inability to use insulin effectively (known as insulin resistance) is an underlying cause of metabolic syndrome. Having metabolic syndrome is a predictor of type 2 diabetes, heart and blood vessel disease and stroke.

Blood pressure describes the amount of force exerted on blood vessel walls as the heart pumps blood around the body. High blood pressure is a very common health problem, putting extra strain on the heart, especially if the blood is also thickened by a high glucose content. Reducing the amount of sugar in the diet can improve blood pressure and blood cholesterol levels. Additionally, cutting salt out of the diet, drinking alcohol in moderation and taking regular exercise help to attain healthy blood pressure levels.

A healthier lifestyle brings the following benefits:

- Weight loss helps the body to use insulin and glucose effectively.
- Lower blood glucose levels are reflected in an HbA1c within normal range.
- Healthier blood pressure levels.
- Reduced levels of harmful blood fats, such as cholesterol.
- Potentially reversing prediabetes and type 2 diabetes so glucose-lowering medicines are no longer needed.

Making significant lifestyle changes to prevent or reverse prediabetes and type 2 diabetes takes a huge amount of commitment from the individual, and this is not a quick and easy process. The patient must be in the right mindset to begin a healthier lifestyle to lose weight and exercise regularly in order to maintain lower glucose levels. This will lower risk of prediabetes and type 2 diabetes, and help to reverse these conditions, but if lifestyle changes are not maintained, weight can be regained, blood glucose levels increase once more and prediabetes and type 2 diabetes return.

Weight Loss Surgery

Sometimes, lifestyle changes have only a minimal effect on the body's ability to use insulin because of metabolic syndrome. Weight loss surgery, known medically as bariatric surgery, has been found to be an effective treatment for type 2 diabetes, enabling insulin to work correctly and for blood glucose levels to be within normal range. However, reversal or remission of prediabetes and type 2 diabetes is not permanent if the individual does not follow treatment advice. Some patients have had surgery to reduce the size of their stomach so that it accepts less food, but then, after some initial weight loss, they have regained weight by regularly eating ice cream and full-fat coffees in addition to their advised small, regular portion diet (Wilson 2022).

Weight loss surgery is considered when a patient's body mass index measurement is above 40. It is now estimated that a quarter of all adults fall into the classification of being obese; in addition, 42% of men and 33% of women are overweight (National Institute for Care Excellence, NICE 2024).

One in six beds in the NHS is currently occupied by a patient with type 1 or type 2 diabetes. The health of more than two million morbidly obese people could be improved by bariatric surgery; this would include the reversal of 40,000 cases of type 2 diabetes, along with 5000 cases of heart disease (NICE 2024).

In the UK, the annual cost of treating health conditions exacerbated by obesity is estimated to be at least £98 billion. This figure includes the costs to the NHS, social care and the impact on productivity (Institute for Global Insights 2023).

There are two types of bariatric surgery: one restricts the size of the stomach, and so slows down digestion so that the patient retains a sense of fullness for longer; the second procedure removes a section of the digestive tract, reducing calorie absorption. Although it is clear that weight loss surgery reduces the quantity of food that can be ingested, without significant diet and exercise changes, surgery becomes far less effective, and in some cases, binge eating still continues (Wilson 2022; Niego et al. 2007).

Bariatric surgery has been used to treat obesity for many years. It has been shown that following surgery, plasma glucose levels return to normal for more than 80% of patients (Keidar 2011). However, this type of surgery decreases life expectancy for morbidly obese patients with a body mass index above 60 (Schauer et al. 2015).

Following surgery procedures for weight loss, blood glucose levels return to normal, despite the fact there is no weight loss. This is due to the reduced amount of food that the stomach has to digest, allowing available insulin to work unhindered by a quantity of starchy carbohydrates.

Although bariatric surgery is usually successful, it has been shown that 95 percent of morbidly obese patients do not lose a substantial amount of weight after one year, due to continuing to overeat, coupled with a lack of exercise and following a healthy diet (Tsai and Wadden 2005; Buchwald et al. 2004).

Reversing Type 2 Diabetes with Bariatric Surgery

Sticking to a recommended diet of small but regular portions of food following surgery, combined with exercise, is essential. Research with 240 morbidly obese patients found that 80% of them became diabetes-free following weight loss surgery and sticking to lifestyle recommendations. This produced an average 60% weight loss (an estimated 44 kg). Patients with type 2 diabetes for less than 5 years achieved the best results and were more likely to have a reversal of their type 2 diabetes (Schauer et al. 2015).

A 10-year follow-up study with 268 participants found that 97% were sustaining normal blood glucose levels for more than a decade (Marinari et al. 2006). It has been shown that when following a healthy lifestyle after surgery, deaths that were attributed to type 2 diabetes had a reduction of up to 92%, but only if the patient adhered to a strict regime (Adams et al. 2007).

The outcome of bariatric surgery varies greatly around the world, with complications of surgery being more significant in less developed countries than in the Western world (Crookes 2006). Poor applications of surgery, such as gastric band slippage, can result in no weight loss, or even weight gain (Crookes 2006; Keidar et al. 2005). Further consequences of poor surgical procedures can result in severe vitamin deficiency, continual vomiting after surgery, pain, loss of bone density, heartburn, constipation, diarrhoea, muscle pain and weakness (Keidar 2011; Crookes 2006).

Weight Loss Drugs

Recently weight lost injections have made the news, with celebrities showing dramatic changes in their shape and clinics around the world having difficulty keeping up with demand. These 'miracle drugs' suppress the appetite to achieve their results; however, they were not initially designed as a weight loss medication.

> By eating less food and not feeling hungry, insulin is able to work well, along the same principle as weight loss surgery, but via a non-invasive method.

The drugs, Ozempic and Mounjaro, are actually medicines to manage type 2 diabetes, growing in popularity with the news that they could also put type 2 diabetes into remission.

- *Ozempic* is an injectable prescription medication that contains the active ingredient *semaglutide*. Ozempic helps the pancreas to produce more insulin, improving blood glucose levels and the management of type 2 diabetes. Ozempic can lead to weight loss; although a different treatment, Wegovy, contains the same weight loss medicine, and is prescribed for this reason for people without type 2 diabetes.
- *Mounjaro* is an injectable prescription medicine used in conjunction with diet and exercise to improve blood glucose levels in adults with type 2 diabetes mellitus.

Ozempic is a prescription-only medicine, so not available for sale over the internet. Some general practitioners (GPs) in the UK are now holding weight loss clinics where they inject the patient every week with Ozempic. Although an injection to help patients lose weight sounds good in principle, as with every medicine Ozempic is not risk-free, and there are negative aspects to be considered.

How Does Ozempic Help Weight Loss?

Ozempic regulates appetite by suppressing hunger. Ozempic, Wegovy and Mounjaro, encourage the pancreas to produce more insulin, slowing down stomach emptying to reduce hunger. Both type 2 diabetes and weight loss can be managed for a maximum of 2 years with Ozempic, the length of time doctors are allowed to prescribe these medicines for. When the stomach has less food, the body tries to get the vital proteins that it needs by reclaiming them from other parts of the body, such as the muscles and bone, ultimately reducing muscle and bone mass.

How Effective Are these Medicines for Weight Loss?

Ozempic treatment results in a 15% loss in bodyweight, while Mounjaro achieves 20%. It is important for patients not to rely on these medicines, as weight loss is not permanent without lifestyle change. Following treatment, appetite returns and some weight is regained, but eating a healthy diet and taking regular exercise prevent a large weight gain. A proportion of weight lost is muscle and bone mass, but after ceasing the treatment the weight regained is gained as fat.

Once appetite returns, more food is eaten at mealtimes, and blood glucose levels increase once more. It is therefore important that a healthy diet without refined carbohydrate is continued to prevent prediabetes becoming type 2 diabetes in the future, or to stop type 2 from returning. Lifestyle change with healthy eating and regular exercise is a far more balanced weight management choice with lasting benefits.

How Long Does Ozempic Take to Work?

Patients usually begin to feel the effects of a reduced appetite and weight loss 2 months after having their first Ozempic injection, which is a weekly process. For patients with type 2 diabetes who take insulin to reduce blood glucose, insulin treatment must be maintained at the same time as having weight loss injections, which regulate appetite and blood glucose. There is an increased risk of blood glucose levels that become too low when patients are eating a reduced diet and taking insulin. It is important for glucose levels to be monitored by the patient and for insulin dosages to be adjusted appropriately to prevent low glucose levels.

What Are the Side Effects of Weight Loss Injections?

Eating much less food can impact on the level of nutrition that the body receives. A highly processed diet is high in calories but low in nutrients, so when taking weight loss injections, the small amount of food ingested must be nutritious.

Ozempic can affect the digestive system, causing vomiting, nausea, diarrhoea or constipation. Because these weight loss medicines encourage the pancreas to produce more insulin, the pancreas can become inflamed, a condition known as pancreatitis. This condition can cause damage to the insulin-producing cells. Although weight is lost, this can be due in part to reduced muscle and bone mass: muscle and bone weigh heavier than fat. The alteration in metabolism that is brought about by taking weight loss injections can lead to kidney, liver and gallbladder disease, in addition to an increased risk of thyroid cancer.

Summary

Various cutting-edge treatments and therapies are currently available to control and effectively manage both type 1 and type 2 diabetes, and there are some future developments that have the potential for temporary or complete reversal of the condition.

Excess weight is also associated with reduced insulin sensitivity, increasing the risk of eventual progression to prediabetes and type 2 diabetes, or making it harder to manage these conditions. Reducing bodyweight by 5–7% (around 10–15 pounds for someone who weighs 200 pounds) lowers blood glucose by improving insulin sensitivity. This eases the amount of work the insulin-producing cells have to do, allowing them to produce insulin for longer.

The majority of type 2 diabetes that is associated with obesity could be put into remission or vastly improved with a healthy, unprocessed diet and regular exercise to achieve weight loss, allowing the metabolism of glucose and the correct action of insulin to be achieved. Getting the right support for weight loss is vital for reducing risk of prediabetes and type 2 diabetes.

In this chapter we have seen currently available options, or diabetes solutions that will soon be realistically offered to patients, which can and will make a real difference to the lives of people with this hidden and sometimes difficult-to-control condition.

References

Adams TD, Gress RE, Smith SC et al (2007) Long-term mortality after gastric bypass surgery. N Engl J Med 357:753–761

Bergenstal RM, Tamborlane WV, Ahmann A et al (2010) Effectiveness of sensor-augmented insulin pump therapy in type 1 diabetes. N Engl J Med 263:311–320

Buchwald H, Avidor Y, Brau E et al (2004) Bariatric surgery: a systematic review and meta-analysis. JAMA J Am Med Assoc 292(14):1724–1737

Burgess MR, Mitchell S, Sawyer A (2008) Continuous glucose monitoring: the future of diabetes management. Diabetes Spectr 21(2):112–119

Centre for Disease Control (2004) Diabetes and smoking. https://www.cdc.gov/diabetes/risk-factors/diabetes-and-smoking.html#:~:text=Quitting%20smoking%20also%20helps%20to,people%20quit%20their%20first%20time

Couri CEB, Volterelli JC (2009) Stem cell therapy for diabetes mellitus: a review of recent trials. Diabetol Metab Syndr 16(1):19–22

Crookes PF (2006) Surgical treatment of morbidly obesity. Annu Rev Med 57:243–264

Darraj A (2023) The link between sleeping and type 2 diabetes: a systematic review. Cureus 15(11):e48228. https://pmc.ncbi.nlm.nih.gov/articles/PMC10693913/#:~:text=The%20risk%20of%20type%202,type%202%20diabetes%20%5B16%5D

Diabetes UK (2008) Early identification of type 2 diabetes and the new vascular risk assessment and management programme. Position statement. Diabetes UK, London

Diabetes UK (2025) Prediabetes symptoms and risk reduction. https://www.diabetes.org.uk/about-diabetes/type-2-diabetes/prediabetes#:~:text=Manage%20your%20weight,risk%20of%20type%202%20diabetes

Efrats S (2009) Stem cell therapy for diabetes: stem cell biology and regenerative medicine. Humana Press, Springer Science and Business Media, New York

Fang M, Yong-Guang Y, Zheng H (2024) Current status and challenges of pig-to-human organ xenotransplantation. Sci China Life Sci 67:829–831

Frederickson L (ed) (1995) The insulin pump therapy book. MiniMed Technologies, Los Angeles, pp 3–4

Gabbe SG, Holing E, Temple P et al (2000) Benefits, risks, costs and patient satisfaction associated with pump therapy complicated by type 1 diabetes mellitus. Am J Obstet Gynecol 182(6):1283–1291

Hakim, N.S., Stratta, R.T., Gray, D. (ed)., et al., (2010) Pancreas, islet, and stem cell transplant for diabetes. 2nd Oxford: Oxford University Press

Institute for Global Insights (2023) Unhealthy numbers: the rising cost of obesity in the UK. https://institute.global/insights/public-services/unhealthy-numbers-the-rising-cost-of-obesity-in-the-uk

Kaufman DB, Sutherland DER (2011) Simultaneous pancreas-kidney transplants are appropriate in insulin-treated candidates with uremia regardless of diabetes type. Clin J Am Soc Nephrol 6(5):957–959

Keidar A (2011) Bariatric surgery for type 2 diabetes reversal: the risk. Diabetes Care 34(2):S361–S367

Keidar A, Szold A, Carmon et al (2005) Band slippage after laparoscopic adjustable gastric banding: etiology and treatment. Surg Endosc 19:262–267

Khan FA (ed) (2011) Stem cell technology: principles and practice, 2012 edn. Springer, London

Klondoff DC, Buckingham B, Christiansen JS et al (2011) Continuous glucose monitoring: an Endocrine Society clinical practice guideline. J Clin Endocrinol Metab 96(10):296–279

Knoll GA, Nichol G (2003) Dialysis, kidney transplantation, or pancreas transplantation for patients with diabetes mellitus and renal failure: a decision analysis of treatment options. Clin J Am Soc Nephrol 14(2):500–515

Marinari GM, Papadia FS, Briatore L (2006) Type 2 diabetes and weight loss following biliopancreatic diversion for obesity. Obes Surg 16:1440–1444

NDST (2005) National Diabetes Support Team factsheet no. 10: working together to reduce the length of stay for people with diabetes. National Diabetes Support Team, London

NICE (2024) Press release: NICE updates—Weight loss surgery criteria for people with type 2 diabetes. nice.org.uk/cg190

Niego SH, Kofman MD, Weiss JJ et al (2007) Binge eating in the bariatric surgery population: a review of the literature. Int J Eat Disord 404:349–359

Pickup JC (2009) Insulin pump therapy and continuous glucose monitoring. Oxford University Press, Oxford

Robertson RP, Holman TV, Genuth S (1998) Pancreas transplantation for type 1 diabetes—a summation. J Clin Endocrinol Metabol 83(6):1868–1874

Ryan EA, Paty BW, Senior PA et al. (2005) Five-year follow-up after clinical islet transplantation. Diabetes 54(7):2060–2069. https://pubmed.ncbi.nlm.nih.gov/15983207/

Sampaio MS, Hung-Tien K, Bunnapradist S (2011) Outcomes of simultaneous pancreas-kidney transplantation in type 2 diabetic recipients. Clin J Am Soc Nephrol 6(5):1198–1206

Schauer PR, Burguera B, Ikramuddin S et al (2015) Effect of laparoscopic roux-en Y gastric bypass on type 2 diabetes mellitus. Ann Surg 238:467–484. (discussion 84–85)

Skyler JS (2000) The economic burden of diabetes and the benefits of improved glycaemic control: the potential role of a continuous glucose monitoring system. Diab Technol Ther 2(1):S7–S11

Sutherland DER, Gruessner RWG (1997) Current status of pancreas transplantation for the treatment of type 1 diabetes mellitus. Clin Diabetes 15:152–156

Sutherland DER, Gruessner RWG (2001) Pancreas transplantation for treatment of diabetes mellitus. World J Surg 25:487–496

Tattersall R (1995) Pancreatic organotherapy for diabetes 1889–1921. History 39:288–316

The Diabetes Control and Complications Trial (DCCT) Research Group (1993) The effect of intensive treatment of diabetes on the development and treatment and progression of long-term complications in insulin-dependent diabetes mellitus. N Engl J Med 329:977–1034

The Diabetes Control and Complications Trial Research Group (1996) Lifetime benefits and costs of intensive therapy as practised in the DCCT. J Am Med Assoc 276:1409–1415

The Diabetes Research and Wellness Foundation (2023) Oxford team begin pioneering human trial of stem cell-derived islet transplants for type 1 diabetes. https://www.drwf.org.uk/news-and-events/news/oxford-team-begin-pioneering-human-trial-of-stem-cell-derived-islet-transplants-for-type-1-diabetes/#:~:text=The%20

UK%20arm%20of%20international,the%20Oxford%20Islet%20Transplant%20Programme

Totey S, Deb KD (2010) Stem cell technology: basics and applications. McGraw Hill Professional, New York

Tsai AG, Wadden TA (2005) Systematic review: an evaluation of major commercial weight loss programmes in the United States. Ann Intern Med 142:56–66

Venstrom JM, McBride MA, Rother et al (2003) Survival after pancreas transplantation in patients with diabetes and preserved kidney function. JAMA 29(210):2817–2823

Walsh J, Roberts R (1999) Pumping insulin: everything in a book for successful use of an insulin pump. Torrey Pines Press, London

Wang X, Metzger DL, Meloche M et al (2012) Generation of transplantable beta cells for patient-specific cell therapy. Int J Endocrinol 2012:414812, 7 pages. https://doi.org/10.1155/2012/414812

Wass, J.A.H., Stewart, P.M., Amiel, S.A., et al. (2011) Oxford textbook of endocrinology and diabetes. Oxford: Oxford University Press, 1856

Wilson VL (2003) Insulin pump therapy: the patient's perspective. Diabetes Primary Care 5(3):132–136

Wilson VL (2005) Insulin pump therapy (CSII). In: Structured patient education in diabetes: report from the Patient Education Working Group. Department of Health/Diabetes UK, London, pp 43–44

Wilson VL (2022) Psychology in diabetes care and practice. Routledge, London/New York, p 135

Wilson VL, Davis JM (2004) NICE: the way forward with insulin pumps. Diabetes Primary Care 6(2):72–76

World Health Organisation (2011) Diabetes factsheet number 312. World Health Organisation, Geneva

9

Global Disparities in Diabetes Care

Type 2 diabetes is currently the fourth main cause of death in developing countries, with the number of people with this condition growing at a faster rate than ever before. With its more prominent and severe symptoms, it is far easier to detect type 1 diabetes, while type 2 diabetes can remain undetected for more than a decade (Diabetes UK 2008). It is therefore very difficult to estimate the number of people worldwide that currently have type 2. As an example, the number of cases in 1985 was estimated to be 30 million and by the year 2000, this estimate had risen to over 150 million; by 2011, the estimated number of type 2 diagnoses worldwide had risen to in excess of 312 million people—12 million more than the estimates up to the year 2025 had predicted (World Health Organisation 2011).

The majority of type 2 diabetes is associated with obesity and consequently, with metabolic factors associated with excess weight. Around the world, it is estimated that 589 million adults currently have diagnosed type 1 or type 2 diabetes, this number having quadrupled in the last 35 years (World Health Organisation 2024).

Due to the slow onset of type 2 diabetes, 50% of people don't know they have it, and in some countries, this is as much as 80%; it is estimated that up to 90% of people who go on to develop type 2 diabetes are classified as obese (WHO 2011).

V. Wilson, *Diabetes Ancient and Modern*, Hippocrates,
https://doi.org/10.1007/978-3-032-12454-8_9

Prevalence (Occurrence)

There are now harsh inequalities in diabetes care. It is the case that in 2022, around 450 million people aged 30 and above had untreated diabetes, with 90% of these people living in less prosperous countries (WHO 2024). Significant differences in diabetes occurrence have been seen across the world, with rates escalating by around 20% among adults aged 18 and above in the South-East Asian and the Eastern Mediterranean Regions. These, together with the African Region, have the lowest access to diabetes treatments: at least 4 in 10 people have no medication to treat high glucose levels (WHO 2024).

What Are the Reasons for These Inequalities?

As rural cultures move to greater industrialisation, and people move to find work, population densities in towns and cities increase. This allows Westernisation, with multinational corporations finding a readily available audience for their products. As profit is the major driving force rather than quality and healthy food, high-fat, high-sugar, high-calorie products have flooded the market and are readily available. As obesity increases, so does a sedentary lifestyle with little or no exercise. This creates a path to prediabetes (high blood glucose levels that are not yet elevated enough to be type 2), and type 2 diabetes, as obesity is a major contributing factor.

An older population means accessibility to food is more restricted as smaller shops don't favour fresh produce as it has a limited shelf life. With populations moving into the towns and cities, there are fewer rural farm workers, and consequently less fresh food is produced. This impacts the traditional lifestyle and dietary patterns, in many cases from healthy unprocessed products to unhealthy highly processed foods containing quantities of fat and sugar. All these factors combine to create a perfect storm for diabetes onset.

> Foods that are 'low fat' tend to be higher in sugar to boost the flavour. Foods and drinks that manufacturers know are unhealthy and high in sugar are marketed as a 'fast energy boost' (increasing blood glucose quickly) because they have no other value in the diet.

Children and Young Adults with Type 2 Diabetes

It is now the case that children as young as 4–5 years of age are classed as being obese; in 2017, 30% of children aged 2–15 were overweight, with 17% being obese (Department of Health 2018). Children who eat 600–700 calories per day in sugary snacks risk developing prediabetes, type 2 diabetes and attention deficit hyperactivity disorder—ADHD (Archer 2014).

With children often leading sedentary lifestyles, frequently playing computer games or watching television, obesity and associated type 2 diabetes will continue to escalate. Type 2 diabetes has been diagnosed in children for over two decades, with over a million new cases of the condition being diagnosed per year in the United States alone, but the developing world is also affected by this escalating epidemic.

In 2021, estimated rates of type 2 diabetes in children and young people reached suggest around 41,600 new cases globally. Germany and the United Kingdom have low rates of type 2 diabetes in non-Hispanic white youths, while the United States, India and China have some of the highest rates (Perng et al. 2023).

The Dominance of Sugar

In the 1700s, sugar was known as white gold because it was so expensive and even by the 1900s, it was still a luxury only afforded and eaten by the wealthy, where sugar was kept under lock and key. Sugar became more widely available with the increase in sugar beet and sugar cane production. In the1940s, sugar formed one quarter of the foods we ate. It now forms a staggering three quarters of our diet (Department of Health 2018). In the UK, by the 1960s the average person ate 68 kg (150 pounds) of sugar per year (Wilson 2021).

Today, access to sugar creates the "Malnutrition of affluence" (Yudkin 2016).

We now consume 20 times more sugar than our ancestors did 300–400 years ago (Wilson 2021). Sugar is more addictive than nicotine, alcohol, morphine or heroin, having a similar effect on the brain. Manufacturers use sugar in their products because people crave sugar, as it's addictive. It is also a cheap ingredient, which bulks and preserves foods, meaning that fewer of the more expensive ingredients need to be added.

Insulin enables fat to be stored by the body, and excess sugar is stored as fat.

Sugar has no nutritional value and the body uses sugar as an instant source of energy, which rapidly increases blood glucose levels. This abnormal imbalance can become toxic at high levels, making it difficult for body systems to work correctly.

Sugar causes the body to release a hormone (ghrelin) that makes us feel hungry and promotes fat storage; it also decreases another hormone (leptin) which promotes the burning of fat for energy (Wilson 2021).

As the world has lived for more than a generation with easy access to sugar, pancreatic islets cells that produce insulin are worked harder and consequently wear out sooner. This increases the likelihood of prediabetes and type 2 diabetes at an earlier age; the likelihood of developing type 2 significantly increases after the age of 45 years (Diabetes UK 2024).

The UK has one of the highest rates of sugar consumption in the world. The increased risk of developing cancers of the pancreas, breast and large intestine are considerably higher in individuals who eat a diet high in sugar and calories, compared to those who consume a healthy, low sugar diet (Romieu et al. 2024; Michaud et al. 2002; Franceschi et al. 2001). In the past 100 years, world sugar production has increased 25-fold (Wilson 2021).

Access to Diabetes Care

There are a number of factors that affect the availability of and accessibility to diabetes care around the world. These include political will, as some countries spend more on military funding than healthcare; whether a country can physically afford healthcare treatments; social structures—those who are able to pay for their treatment will receive it, while those who cannot pay go without it; quality of care depending on the infrastructure in place, such as diabetes-trained medical staff with access to technological advancements, and educational resources, including health education.

Political influence in some countries and regions within these countries focusses on their own agenda which might not include adequate distribution of medical resources to the general population. Lower income countries do not have the budget to spend on diabetes essentials, such as insulin, syringes and glucose testing equipment, let alone more advanced technologies, such as insulin pumps and continuing glucose monitoring systems.

The relationship between diabetes, poor economy and societal poverty is well documented. For those who pay for their own diabetes care, cost of necessary diabetes supplies, such as insulin, combined with self-funding treatment options, such as insulin pump therapy, creates barriers for those with low incomes, leading to prioritising what can be afforded. This ultimately has consequences regarding being able to manage diabetes effectively.

Regardless of the cost of insulin and diabetes equipment, the key aspect of care has to be its delivery by appropriately trained staff. Poorer nations have a greater disparity between a minority of well-educated people and the rest of the nation. Those within the medical profession are highly educated and consequently in demand, meaning that many seek employment overseas in better-paid jobs following their medical training. This leaves behind those that are less well-educated to cover all aspects of diabetes medical care, often with a higher ratio of patient-to-staff numbers when compared to a Western nation. The retention of staff is not only a problem for poorer nations, but also richer ones too, as specially trained personnel are at a premium and can consequently sell their skills to the highest bidder.

Urban and Rural Disparities

In addition to these issues, there are discrepancies between people with diabetes who live in towns and cities compared with those who live in rural areas, and tribal racism which can create cultural and language barriers. These factors each contribute to a disparity in diabetes care worldwide, creating a healthcare lottery regarding available diabetes-prevention education; prediabetes and type 2 diabetes diagnoses and treatment outcomes, combined with a differing life expectancy.

Cheaper Junk Foods

A main contributor towards the global type 2 diabetes epidemic, and especially in low- to middle-income countries, is the widespread availability of highly processed 'junk' foods that are cheaper than healthier foods such as lean meat, vegetables, fruits and wholegrain bread. There has been an unhealthy change in favour of diets that are high in refined carbohydrates, fat, sugar, salt and calories, in association with little or no exercise. These factors have been mentioned earlier as a leading cause of obesity, prediabetes and type 2 diabetes.

> Empty calories, such as those found in canned fizzy drinks, contribute nothing to daily nutrition. Drinking three 330 mL cans of these drinks each day equals approximately 150,000 empty calories per year, the equivalent of a man's recommended daily intake of 2500 calories for 2 months.

The World Health Organisation reported an alarming increase in type 2 diabetes over the past three decades in association with economic hardship, marketing and availability of unhealthy food, obesity and insufficient exercise (WHO 2024). These factors have had a particular impact on rates of type 2 diabetes in low- to middle-income countries, putting huge pressure on available healthcare provision (Hu 2011). The increase in adult type 2 diabetes between 1990 and 2022 has seen a soaring trend, while access to healthcare remains limited.

Westernised nations consistently have the same multinational corporations selling foods right across their countries. To keep profits high all foodstuffs other than fresh fruit and vegetables tend to be mass produced, with many of these being highly processed. Inevitably, this usually means high sugars in various forms. Sugar has no nutritional value, yet sugar is often added to baby foods to add calories, rather than nutrients (Thomas 2025), hooking the child on sweet foods from an early age.

> As we know sugars are easily converted to energy, while carbohydrates take longer for the body to digest. The body stores this excess energy in the form of various fats, which in turn leads to type 2 diabetes.

Less-developed countries have greater access to sugars now than ever before, and although these countries tend to be more loosely based on agriculture, those living in the towns and cities have greater access to poor dietary foods. Ironically these nations tend to sell their food produce to the richer nations to generate income, rather than eating a better home-grown diet.

Access to Insulin

In 2010, out of 120 countries, only 48 had consistent supplies of insulin, but this figure was only estimated for urban areas (Gill et al. 2010). The majority of people with type 2 diabetes do not immediately treat this condition with insulin, although when oral blood glucose-lowering medication (such as metformin) begins to fail, insulin is required. For people who need insulin, in Africa and Asia whether type 2 or type 1 (which is also increasing in number) availability is outpaced by demand, although insulin is more accessible in urban areas than rural (Mbanya and Mba 2021).

Industrialised Western nations have greater access to diabetes treatment, including insulin, syringes, insulin pumps and consumables and blood glucose testing equipment. This represents a lesser percentage of an individual's annual income when compared to that of some African countries. The cost of insulin alone in Mali, for example, was 39% of a family income in the year 2000—this does not include syringes to deliver the insulin, or blood-testing equipment to monitor diabetes self-management. Despite the fact that the cost of insulin is subsidised in some African countries, the cost to a family still represents a significant burden (Walker et al. 2023).

However, the cost of diabetes healthcare in some Westernised countries can also be daunting for the individual. In the United States, where healthcare costs are covered by private medical insurance, premiums have escalated to such an extent that diabetes self-care has priced itself out of the market (Hassan et al. 2024). The average price of insulin increased threefold between 2002 and 2013 (Hua et al. 2016).

Nearly half of people with diabetes in the USA reported that they had not had essential diabetes care at some point due to the cost involved (Lardiera 2018). Again, this includes an annual review with a diabetes consultant or diabetic eye screening, rather than insulin syringes, or blood glucose testing equipment.

In the UK, the NHS covers the cost of diabetes care, although patients with type 2 diabetes must fund their own glucose self-monitoring systems.

Due to the lack of competitive insulin production, the two main insulin manufacturers—Eli Lilley and Novo Nordisk—have recently increased their prices and their possible profits, reflecting on availability in poorer nations. There are various campaigns around the world calling for cheaper insulin and improved accessibility (Hua et al. 2016).

Complications and Mortality

Without regular access to necessary insulin, chronic complications of high blood glucose levels are inevitable. The disparity between lower and higher income countries is reflected in healthcare provision. Poorer nations lack the infrastructure with regard to medical technology and facilities, comprehensive patient education and health beliefs. Limited healthcare budgets mean prioritisation of immediate health conditions such as AIDS and malaria, rather than the slow progression of type 2 diabetes and chronic complications.

Around 80% of people with type 2 diabetes live in low- to middle-income countries (International Diabetes Federation 2019), with many more undiagnosed. This escalating figure will continue to climb as more people move into towns and cities (Hu 2011), increasing access to an unhealthy diet of processed and fast foods, increasing salt and sugar in the diet, combined with a multitude of additives and preservatives. This change in behaviour is associated with a more sedentary lifestyle with little or no exercise.

Low to middle healthcare systems are already dealing with localised issues such as infectious diseases like dengue fever and tuberculosis, which are more common in low- to middle-income countries, as well as pneumonia (van Crevel et al. 2017; Zar et al. 2013). Any infection causes blood glucose levels to rise as the body fights the disease, meaning that deaths related to a combination of disease and already high glucose are common.

On top of this, health services have to accommodate treatment of chronic diabetes complications. There is little research concerning the impact of chronic complications in low-income countries (Almirall et al. 2017; Shen et al. 2017; IDF 2016). However, a causal link between high blood glucose levels and the development of complications is well-established (Diabetes Control and Complications Trial 1993).

More developed nations screen for diabetic complications such as cardiovascular (heart), kidney disease and retinopathy (eye) disease, which is not carried out to such an extent in lower income countries. Undiagnosed type 2 diabetes has a significant impact on the heart and circulatory system. In less developed countries heart disease is more likely to develop in those with untreated and undiagnosed type 2 diabetes (Fowler 2011). High blood pressure and arterial disease also increase the likelihood of stroke (Van Dieren et al. 2010).

Rates of depression are also high in wealthier countries, but as a major contributor to high glucose levels, increased rates of depression in poorer countries are rarely recognised and treated. Due to the lack of detection of chronic complications, when they are recognised, they are more severe, increasing mortality rates (IDF 2016; Thomas et al. 2016; Mendenhall et al. 2017).

Foot Disease

Diabetic foot disease is the most common reason for amputation besides accident or injury, and this outcome is strongly linked with poor access to necessary and preventative healthcare. Worldwide, diabetic nerve disease and poor circulation cause foot ulcers and infection, leading to a lower limb amputation every 30 seconds (International Diabetes Federation 2025), with the risk of amputation for people with diabetes being 25 times greater than for those without the condition (IDF 2025). This is the case because an estimated 183 million people across the globe have diabetic foot disease (Armstrong et al. 2017).

These eventual amputations begin with a diabetic foot ulcer in 85% of cases (Pecoraro et al. 1990). This has a major impact on mortality, especially in lower income countries where sepsis and access to antibiotic drug treatments, slow healing due to diabetes and heat and humidity can increase the likelihood of infection.

Following lower limb amputation, further health requirements include assistive technologies such as crutches, wheelchairs and prosthetic limbs. However, according to the WHO, only around 5–15% of patients in low-income countries who need assistive technologies receive them (WHO 2010). Chronic complications ultimately result in a lesser quality of life for the patient (Khunkaew et al. 2019) and an associated increase in mortality rates (Iversen et al. 2009).

Eye Disease

There is an estimated threefold difference between visual loss in South Asian, North African and Middle Eastern populations compared with Western sub-Saharan Africa.

Globally, 43 million people have little to no sight; 552 million have visual impairment and 510 million people have impaired close vision: approximately 90% of these individuals live in low- to middle-income countries (Burton et al. 2021).

In many cases, vision can be restored with available treatment and care. These include:

- 160 million cases of diabetic retinopathy among 463 million patients with diabetes (Burton et al. 2021).

Retinopathy leads to blood vessel leakage from the tiny vessels at the back of the eyes, and promotes new abnormal blood vessel growth. High glucose levels increase pressure in the eyes, leading to fluid build-up which in turn makes protein stick to the lens of the eye, eventually leading to cataract and blindness. Retinopathy in patients with diabetes is the leading cause of blindness in developing countries (Van Dieren et al. 2010).

Those in rural communities with chronic complications are significantly affected far more than those in urban areas. The increasing numbers of people with type 2 diabetes and their complications place a strain on healthcare systems.

Treatment Rates

In lower to middle-income countries, a significant number of people with diabetes remain untreated and this number has increased since 1990 due to population growth, migration into towns and cities, and cost of treatment. Even in higher income countries, inequalities still exist based on cost of care, and genetic factors affecting ethnic populations.

Early detection of type 2 diabetes is vital to reduce the chance of developing complications in the future. There are currently millions who are undiagnosed worldwide, in both rich and poor countries alike. This only goes to show how great a problem diabetes has become. It is not an exaggeration to call type 2 diabetes a worldwide epidemic with a significant proportion of medical costs firmly attributed to treating accompanying chronic complications, many of which lead to an early death.

Discrimination and Marginalisation

When it comes to diabetes care, certain populations experience discrimination brought about by a number of social factors. Diabetes disproportionately affects populations and cultures who are excluded from mainstream society and lack access to resources due to factors such as poverty, ethnicity, race, gender, disability or sexual orientation. There are often multiple factors leading to poor diabetes self-management, a higher rate of complications and reduced quality of life, each exacerbating these risks (Martinez-Cruz et al. 2025).

Psychosocial factors such as low self-esteem, housing uncertainty, doubts over providing food for the family and low incomes each play their part in preventing these individuals from accessible medical care and necessary medications, especially under a health insurance scheme. Religious and cultural factors, fat shaming at having caused type 2 diabetes—stigma or being treated differently because of it, exclusion surrounding having diabetes and poor diabetes self-knowledge also reduce the ability to cope with and manage the condition effectively.

Certain minority groups, such as those with disability, mental health problems or ethnicity often face discrimination and receive an insufficient level of diabetes care. Health education requirements need to match the individual's needs; if an individual is blind or deaf, faces linguistic obstacles or other psychosocial barriers which prevent good diabetes self-care, motivation from health professionals, family and friends are also key. To be able to participate in learning about and carrying out necessary diabetes self-care, accessible and understandable healthcare appointments and health education must take account of these factors so that understanding is ensured.

Other influencing factors affecting diabetes management concern the community's access to nutritional food; urbanisation of areas with very little green space; constricted living accommodation and space which reflects on wellbeing and the impact that the local environment has on the individual.

What Can Be Done About These Disparities?

The World Health Organization (WHO) is working on international coherent plans, such as the Global Diabetes Compact, aiming to reduce the risk of diabetes, and ensuring that all people who are diagnosed with the condition have access to reasonable, comprehensive, affordable and quality treatment and care. The work undertaken as part of the Global Diabetes Compact will also support the prevention of type 2 diabetes from obesity, unhealthy diet and physical inactivity (WHO 2025).

It is essential that insulin is made continuously available for those who need it around the world, along with syringes and blood glucose testing equipment.

Diabetes education must be tailored to the specific needs of the individual, taking into account patient empowerment—meaning the perceived ability to carry out self-care tasks, oblivious of health status; ethnicity and language barriers; socioeconomic and financial considerations; and geographic isolation.

Conclusion

A fundamental increase in type 2 diabetes is sweeping the world as developing nations are subject to Westernisation and urbanisation. This brings with it the twin evils of high sugar and processed foods as populations adopt a Westernised diet which increases levels of obesity and associated type 2 diabetes. This course is likely to continue without significant intervention.

References

Almirall J, Serra-Prat M, Bolibar I et al (2017) Risk factors for community-acquired pneumonia in adults: a systematic review of observational studies. Respiration 94:299–311

Archer D (2014) ADHD and refined sugar: can refined sugar trigger ADHD?. https://www.psychologytoday.com/us/blog/reading-between-the-headlines/201404/adhd-and-refined-sugar

Armstrong DG, Boulton AJ, Bus SA (2017) Diabetic foot ulcers and their recurrence. N Engl J Med 376:2367–2375

Burton MJ, Ramke J, Marques AP et al (2021) The Lancet Global Health Commission on global eye health: vision beyond 2020. Lancet Glob Health 9(4):e489–e551

Department of Health (2018) Health survey for England, 2017: adult and child obesity. https://ww.healthsurvey.hscic.gov.uk/media/78619/HSE17-adult-child-BMI-rep.pdf

Diabetes Control and Complications Trial (DCCT) Research Group (1993) The effect of intensive treatment of diabetes on the development and treatment and progression of long-term complications in insulin-dependent diabetes mellitus. N Engl J Med 329:977–034

Diabetes UK (2008) Early identification of type 2 diabetes and the new vascular risk assessment and management programme. Position statement update. Diabetes UK, London

Diabetes UK (2024) Type 2 diabetes prevention week 2024: action needed to tackle rising number of type 2 cases in under 40s. https://www.diabetes.org.uk/about-us/news-and-views/diabetes-prevention-week-2024-action-needed-tackle-rising-type-2-cases#:~:text=Colette%20Marshall%2C%20Chief%20Executive%20of,but%20also%20the%20next%20generation

Fowler MJ (2011) Microvascular and macrovascular complications of diabetes. Clin Diabetes 29(3):116–122

Franceschi S, Dal Maso L, Augustin L et al (2001) Dietary glycaemic load and colorectal cancer risk. Ann Oncol 12(2):173–178

Gill GV, Yudkin JS, Keen H et al (2010) The insulin dilemma in resource-limited countries. A way forward? Published online by Springer. www.haiweb.org/medicine-prices/07072010/Global_briefing_note_FINAL.pdf

Hassan S, Gujral UP, Quarells RC et al (2024) Global inequality in diabetes 3: disparities in diabetes prevalence and management by race and ethnicity in the USA: defining a path forwards. Lancet Diabetes Endocrinol 11(7):509–524

Hu FB (2011) Globalization of diabetes: the role of diet, lifestyle, and genes. Diabetes Care 34:1249–1257

Hua X, Carvalho N, Tew M et al (2016) Expenditure and prices of antihyoerglycaemic medications in the United States: 2002–2013. JAMA 315(13):1400–1402

International Diabetes Federation (2016) Diabetes and cardiovascular disease. International Diabetes Federation, Brussels

International Diabetes Federation (2019) IDF diabetes atlas, 9th edn. International Diabetes Federation, Brussels

International Diabetes Federation (2025) Complications. https://idf.org/about-diabetes/diabetes-complications/

Iversen MM, Tell GS, Riise T et al (2009) History of foot ulcer increases mortality among individuals with diabetes: ten-year follow-up of the Nord-Trøndelag Health Study, Norway. Diabetes Care 32:2193–2199

Khunkaew S, Fernandez R, Sim J (2019) Health-related quality of life among adults living with diabetic foot ulcers: a meta-analysis. Qual Life Res 28:1413–1427

Lardiera A (2018) Almost half of diabetics skip care because of high cost. Am News. https://www.usnews.com/news/health-care-news/articles/2018-06-18/study-almost-half-of-diabetics-skip-care-because-of-high-cost

Martinez-Cruz MS, Mamasingh N, Alexopoulos A-S et al (2025) The forgotten – overcoming challenges in diabetes care for marginalized populations. 20(5):385–401

Mbanya JC, Mba CM (2021) Centenary of the discovery of insulin: people with diabetes in Africa still have poor access to insulin. EClinicalMedicine. https://www.thelancet.com/journals/eclinm/article/PIIS2589-5370(21)00089-4/fulltext

Mendenhall E, Kohrt BA, Norris SA (2017) Non-communicable disease syndemics: poverty, depression, and diabetes among low-income populations. Lancet 389:951–963

Michaud DS, Liu S, Giovannucci E et al (2002) Dietary sugar, glycaemic load, and pancreatic cancer risk in a prospective study. J Natl Cancer Inst 94(17):1293–1300

Pecoraro RE, Reiber GE, Burgess EM (1990) Pathways to diabetic limb amputation. Basis for prevention. Diabetes Care 13:513–521

Perng W, Conway R, Mayer-Davis E et al (2023) Youth-onset type 2 diabetes: the epidemiology of an awakening epidemic. Diabetes Care 46(3):490–499

Romieu I, Lazcano-Ponce E, Sanchez-Zamorano. LM et al (2024) Carbohydrates and the risk of breast cancer among Mexican women. Cancer Epidemiol Biomarkers Prev 13(8):1283–1289

Shen Y, Cai R, Sun J et al (2017) Diabetes mellitus as a risk factor for incident chronic kidney disease and end-stage renal disease in women compared with men: a systematic review and meta-analysis. Endocrine 55:66–76

Thomas T (2025) Leading baby food brands making high-sugar meals, study finds. The Guardian. https://www.theguardian.com/society/2025/apr/28/leading-baby-food-brands-making-high-sugar-meals-study-finds

Thomas MC, Cooper ME, Zimmet P (2016) Changing epidemiology of type 2 diabetes mellitus and associated chronic kidney disease. Natl Rev Nephrol 12:73–81

van Crevel R, van de Vijver S, Moore DAJ (2017) The global diabetes epidemic: what does it mean for infectious diseases in tropical countries? Lancet Diabetes Endocrinol 5:457–468

Van Dieren S, Beulens JW, van der Schouw Y (2010) The global burden of diabetes and its complications: an emerging pandemic. Eur J Prev Cardiol 171:S7–S8

Walker AF, Graham S, Maple-Brown L et al (2023) Interventions to address global inequality in diabetes: international progress. Lancet 402(10397):250–264

Wilson VL (2021) How to reduce your child's sugar intake. Little Brown Book Group, London, Robinson

World Health Organisation (2010) Assistive/devices/technologies. World Health Organisation, Geneva

World Health Organisation (2011) Diabetes factsheet number 312. World Health Organisation, Geneva

World Health Organisation (2024). Urgent action needed as global diabetes cases increase four-fold over past decades. https://www.who.int/news/item/13-11-2024-urgent-action-needed-as-global-diabetes-cases-increase-four-fold-over-past-decades#:~:text=The%20number%20of%20adults%20living%20with%20diabetes,in%20The%20Lancet%20on%20World%20Diabetes%20Day

World Health Organisation (2025) The WHO global diabetes compact. https://www.who.int/initiatives/the-who-global-diabetes-compact

Yudkin J (2016) Pure, white and deadly. Penguin Life

Zar HJ, Madhi SA, Aston SJ et al (2013) Pneumonia in low- and middle-income countries: progress and challenges. Thorax 68:1052–1056

Diabetes Timeline

1536 B.C.	*The Ebers papyrus*, in which the Egyptian physician of the Third Dynasty *Hesy-Ra* wrote on excessive thirst and frequent urination, the first mention of symptoms that can be attributed to diabetes.
600 B.C.	The Indian physician *Sushruta* identifies the differences between type 1 and type 2 diabetes, noting that one started quickly, the other slowly. He also noted that urine from people with diabetes tasted sweet, and that this was not the case in someone without diabetes.
470–360 B.C.	*Hippocrates* recognises in his writings that diabetes is a wasting disease associated with frequent urination.
300 B.C.	*Herophilus* of Chalcedon (Greece) is the first to describe the pancreas in a written account. Indian physicians name diabetes *Madhumeha* (honey-like urine).
250 B.C.	The Greek physician *Arateus* defines the outcome of diabetes as *the melting down of flesh and limbs into urine.*
200 B.C.	Written during the Hang Dynasty in ancient China, The *Huang Di Nei Jing (The Yellow Emperor's Classic of Internal Medicine)* gives a description that defines diabetes.
100 A.D.	The physician and anatomist *Rufus of Ephesus* gives the pancreas its name: *pan*—meaning all, and *creas*—meaning flesh.

V. Wilson, *Diabetes Ancient and Modern*, Hippocrates,
https://doi.org/10.1007/978-3-032-12454-8

120 A.D.	*Aretaeus of Cappodocia* (81–138 A.D.) further defined diabetes, using the Greek word for siphon or water pipe to describe the incessant flow of urine in cases of diabetes. He also described the differences between the two separate diseases, diabetes mellitus (with sugar in the urine) and diabetes insipidus (without sugar in the urine).
128–201 A.D.	*Galen* was a Greek physician from Pergamum who gave the description *diarrhoea of the urine* and *the thirsty disease* to describe diabetes.
Fourth–Fifth centuries	*Oribasius* was a Byzantine physician who recognised a type of diabetes that began in childhood. He also suggested a remedy for diabetes that occurred in older, fatter individuals 'to alter the patient's temperament from moist to warm to render the individual lean'.
Sixth century A.D.	*Aetius* was a physician from Amida who would take a blood sample to observe 'the fatness' of a patient's blood (this was later understood to have a higher glucose content than normal).
Sixth century A.D.	*Stephanus* was a Greek physician from Athens who inspected the patients' urine (uroscopy) for properties such as cloudiness, smell, colour, blood and thickness—indicating the presence of glucose.
589–618 A.D.	*Zhen Li-Yan* was a Chinese physician who observed that the dilute urine of people with diabetes tended to be *sweet and without fat.*
752 A.D.	*Wang Tao* documented that the urine of people with diabetes contains sugar in *Wai Tai Mi Yao (A Collection of Diseases*). He advised his patients to pass urine over a wide, flat brick and if ants and flies gathered on the brick, this proved that the insects had found sugar.
Ninth century	*Paul of Aegina* was a Byzantine physician, who called diabetes *dipsacus*—meaning a weakening of the kidneys that could cause dehydration.
865–925 A.D.	*Rhazes*, a renowned Persian physician translated the entire Indian knowledge on diabetes and recommended potential cures for obesity and frequent urination.
932 A.D.	*Isaac Judaeus* documented a book dedicated to nutrition and diet, thought to be the first ever book of this kind.
Died 994 A.D.	*Haly Abbas* was another Persian physician who defined diabetes as an excess of heat in the body, naming this *dysentery of the discrepancy.*

980–1037 A.D.	*Avicenna* was a Persian physician who not only outlined the causes of diabetes, but also mentioned complications including blindness and poor circulation leading to gangrene.
1162–1231	*Abd al-Latif al-Baghdadi* wrote a dedicated treatise on diabetes.
1493–1541	*Paracelsus* was a Swiss physician who considered diabetes to be a serious health problem.
1621–1675	*Thomas Willis* was an English physician who coined the phrase *the pissing evil* to describe diabetes mellitus. In one of his experiments, he evaporated diabetic urine and on tasting it, found it to be sweet.
1682	*Johann Conrad Brunner* observes a great thirst and frequent urination in dogs after having part of their pancreas removed.
1745–1821	*Johann Peter Frank* chemically confirmed the difference between the two conditions, diabetes mellitus and diabetes insipidus calling this type of diabetes 'spurious' as the urine contained no glucose.
1706	*John Rollo*, Surgeon-General to the Royal Artillery, used a restrictive diet to treat a patient with type 1 diabetes.
1774	*Robert Wyatt*, an English physician, concluded from his experiments that the presence of glucose in both blood and urine was a common factor in patients with diabetes.
1776	*Mathew Dobson* confirms similarly to Wyatt that an excessive amount of glucose is present in both the blood and urine of people with diabetes.
1788	*Thomas Cawley*, an anatomist, documented that the post-mortem pancreas of patients with diabetes had an altered appearance to that of a normal pancreas.
1798	*John Rollo* drew the conclusion that high levels of glucose resulted in cataracts and autonomic nerve damage affecting digestion, the genitals, the bladder and kidneys.
1815	*Eugene Chevreuil* was a chemist who recognised, following chemical experimentation, that the sugar present in a patient with diabetes was in fact glucose.
1818–1876	*Ludwig Traube* showed through experimentation that the amount of carbohydrate eaten appears as a similar amount of glucose in the urine.
1832	*Richard Bright* recognised the importance that the pancreas has in the metabolism of food.

1850	*Piorry* observed that as a large amount of sugar was being passed in the urine, his patients should replace this lost sugar with equally substantial amounts in their diet.
1857	*Claude Bernard* proposed that excess production of glucose in the body is the cause of diabetes.
1864	*Marchal de Calvi* noted the relationship between diabetes as the cause of peripheral neuropathy.
1869	*Paul Langerhans* discovered cells in the pancreas he believed to be lymph glands. These glands were later identified as the insulin-producing cells (islets) of the pancreas which were named after him. *Noyes* reports a case of retinitis in a diabetic patient in the same year.
1871	*Bouchardat* notices that in association with the Franco-Prussian War, rationing caused glucose to disappear from the urine of patients with diabetes.
1803–1873	*Justus von Liebig* shows the breakdown of foods in human metabolism which then creates energy.
1874	*Kussmaul* describes the altered breathing as 'air hunger' in cases of diabetic ketoacidosis.
1876	*Étienne Lancereaux* describes the clinical differences between type 1 and type 2 diabetes.
1884	*Althaus* notices that the severe peripheral nerve pain in his patients' feet and legs is worse at night than during the day. *Bouchard* observes the lack of knee jerk reflexes in patients with severe peripheral nerve damage in diabetes.
1885	*Frederick Pavy* recognised the association between high blood and urine glucose levels and peripheral nerve damage.
1887	*Pryce* notes that a reduction in blood supply in the lower legs is a major contributing factor in diabetic leg ulceration and gangrene.
1889	*Joseph von Mering* and *Oskar Minowski* concluded that the pancreas is key in the development of diabetes, but uncertainty still remained over the importance of pancreatic secretions, and whether they regulated glucose levels, or if this was a role of the kidneys.
1890	*Charcot* documented the effect of peripheral nerve damage on the bones and joints in people with diabetes.

Purdy expressed the view that almost every person with diabetes had some degree of nerve damage, and that it was unusual to see a patient who did not.

1892 *Laguesse* observed at autopsy the minute structural deterioration of the pancreatic tissue at cell level in diabetic patients.

Battistini and *Capparelli* try to cure diabetes by injecting pancreatic powder extracts.

1893 *Dr. P. Watson Williams* in Bristol, England, performed the first pancreas transplant from sheep to human on December 20, which proved unsuccessful.

1898 *Eliott Joslin* proposed opium as a treatment for diabetes.

1900 *Bayliss* and *Starling* identified the chemical messengers that regulate secretions from the endocrine glands.

Tests are developed which can detect glucose in urine.

1901 *Eugene Opie* observed a link between the onset of diabetes and the failure of the islets of Langerhans in the production of insulin.

1906 *Wilhelm Heiberg* developed a method for counting the islets of Langerhans, proving that they are limited in diabetic patients.

1907 *Rennie* and *Fraser* administered their pancreatic extract to five patients with type 1 diabetes, although there was no observable change in blood glucose levels.

1909 *Jean de Meyer* introduced the name 'insulin'.

1910 *Joseph Pratt* published 'The relation of the pancreas to diabetes' in the Journal of the American Medical Association.

1911 *Georg Zuelzer* gave diabetic dogs his pancreatic extract (*acomatrol*), with limited success.

1912 *Ernest Scott* was a researcher who observed that removing or tying off the pancreatic duct in dogs attracted flies to the animals' urine. He had some success in treating dogs with pancreatic extract, although he did not recognise the importance of this finding.

1913 *John Macleod* was a professor and diabetes specialist at the University of Toronto who wrote *Diabetes: Its Pathological Physiology*.

1916 *Edward Sharpey-Schäfer* used the name *insuline* to describe a hormone made by the pancreas that reduced the amount of glucose in the blood.

1917 *Elliot Joslin* was a diabetes specialist who had seen in excess of 1000 cases of the condition. He wrote *The Treatment of Diabetes Mellitus* based on his knowledge and observations of his patients.

1919 *Frederick Allen* was a diabetes specialist who suggested a starvation diet for his patients with diabetes, writing *Total Dietary Regulations in the Treatment of Diabetes.*

1921 *Nicolas Paulesco* was a contemporary of Banting and Best in developing an injectable and effective blood glucose-lowering secretion. He published his work using *pancreatine*, but then discovered that his rivals had also achieved success with their discovery *isletin.*

1922 *Leonard Thompson* was given isletin by John Macleod and became the first person to have their type 1 diabetes treated in this way. The term 'insulin' described a pure pancreatic extract, and this was used instead of isletin. Macleod patented insulin to Toronto University, and the pure extract was then mass-produced by Eli Lilly.

1923 *Banting* and *Macleod* are honoured for their discovery of insulin, receiving the Nobel Prize (although this was the work of Banting and Best, the discovery was made in Macleod's laboratory). Banting shared his prize money with Banting, while it was suggested that Macleod share his with chemist, *James Collip.*

J.C. Meakins produce insulin at the Edinburgh Royal Infirmary, using it to treat patients in the Diabetes Department.

Insulin dosage becomes standardised into units.

The *Nordisk* manufacturer is established in Denmark.

1924 *Frederick Charles Pybus* an English surgeon, attempted to graft pancreatic tissue to cure diabetes.

1925 It is first suggested that insulin could perhaps be inhaled by aerosol.

1926 *John Abel* purified insulin and discovered that it has a translucent structure.

1927 *Elliot Joslin* the diabetes specialist devised a diabetes diet treatment for both type 1 and type 2 diabetes that was low in carbohydrates.

1930 Chronic complications of diabetes are found to be due to the lasting damage to cells and tissues caused by high blood glucose levels.

1934 *H.G. Wells* the science fiction writer, and *R.D. Lawrence* (both persons with type 2 diabetes) formed the British Diabetic Association as a support network for others with the condition.

Joslin observed a causal relationship between eye and kidney disease, and diabetes.

1935 *Harold Himsworth* recognised that the two types of diabetes have different reactions to insulin. Type 1 diabetes is due to a lack of insulin, where there is insulin sensitivity; in type 2 diabetes there is often too much insulin being produced, although the tissues of the body lack sensitivity to insulin so that it cannot work correctly.

1936 *Protamine* zinc insulin was introduced by Nordisk with components that delay the insulin working time.

1938 *Allen Whipple* documented the successful treatment of low blood glucose levels after giving the patient glucose.

1940 *Hans Krebs* explained the way in which diabetes develops, identifying the key stages.

1944 Everest the glass maker produced the first glass and stainless steel syringe for insulin administration.

1946 The introduction of *Isophane* insulin (marketed as Insultard) which is designed to be mixed with other insulins to have a working time that covers the peak in blood glucose after meals.

1953 One of the most popular insulins of its time, taken by one third of people around the world with diabetes, *Lente* was introduced by Novo. However, it was not able to be mixed with regular insulins.

1957 *Solomon Berson* and *Rosalyn Yalow* introduce the technique of immunoassay to detect or measure specific proteins. This method could be used to detect insulin in someone's system.

1958 *Marcel Janbon* and *August Loubatieres* find that herbal remedies, such as French lilac (goat's rue) contain *sulfonylureas* that encourage the pancreatic islet cells to produce insulin.

The blood glucose-lowering drugs, *carbutamide, chlopropamide, tolbutamide* and *toldzamide* are first marketed for the treatment of type 2 diabetes.

1959 Metformin is introduced under the marketing name *Glucophage* (sugar-eater) and is used across Europe to treat type 2 diabetes. Although metformin still has some

	toxic effects, its toxicity is lower than other biguanides derived from the same plant sources. These toxic effects meant that the drug was not licensed in the United States of America until 1995.
1960	Physicists *Yalow* and *Berson* prove that obesity prevents insulin from working correctly in cases of type 2 diabetes, even though sufficient insulin is being produced.
	Arnold Kadish introduces the first wearable insulin pump, although it is the size of a small rucksack.
1961	The development of a single-use plastic insulin syringe was introduced by Becton Dickinson.
1963	Insulin pumps are introduced as a treatment for type 1 diabetes.
1966	*Kelly* performs the first complete human pancreas transplant, carried out at the University of Manitoba.
1969	*Dorothy Crowfoot Hodgkin* (Nobel Laureate) describes the structure of insulin.
	Ames Diagnostics produced a portable blood glucose meter, the first to be used in hospital Emergency Departments.
1970	Diabetic eye disease is treated with lasers to treat and delay blindness.
1971	*Anton Clemens* receives the first blood glucose monitor produced by Ames Reflectance for use in his home.
1972	Introduction of the first standardised U100 insulin.
1974	Development of monocomponent (MC) insulin, or single-peak insulin.
	Gérard Slama and colleagues in Paris show that a few days of using an open-loop intravenous insulin infusion pump in type 1 diabetes produces good blood glucose control.
1978	*Pirart* shows that in a 25-year study, small blood vessel complications are common in both type 1 and type 2 diabetes.
1982	*Monocomponent* insulin, which is ultra-pure, is introduced by *Novo.* This insulin has only one component.
1986	The introduction of the insulin pen makes injecting insulin easier for people with diabetes.

1987	Genetically engineered yeast cells enable Novo to produce pure human insulin under laboratory conditions.
1989	*NovoNordisk* is the new name following the merger of *Novo Industri A/S* and *Nordisk Gentofte A/S*. This conglomerate becomes the largest manufacturer of insulin.
1992	Medtronic releases the MiniMed 506 insulin pump.
1993	The Diabetes Control and Complications Trial (DCCT) demonstrated that if type 1 diabetes is well controlled there is a significant reduction in the development of chronic complications.
1994	*Metformin* is sold under the brand name metformin by the Bristol-Myers Squibb pharmaceutical company in the UK.
1996	Lily introduced *Humalog*, a short-acting insulin to reduce the likelihood of low blood glucose levels.
1998	The UK Prospective Diabetes Study (UKPDS) concluded that tighter control of type 2 diabetes leads to reduced rates of eye, kidney and heart disease.
2000	The Dosage Adjustment for Normal Eating (DAFNE) education course was introduced for patients with type 1 diabetes.
2002	Glargine (Lantus) is introduced. This insulin is longer acting with no peak working times.
2003	Insulin pumps were first used in research in the 1970s and 1980s. Modern pumps became smaller and user-friendly in the early 2000s.
2005	The insulin inhaler is introduced (for adults) after approval by the Federal Drugs Administrator in the US.
2006	N.I.C.E. (The National Institute for Health and Clinical Excellence) approved the use of insulin inhalers for both types of diabetes in the UK. The Diabetes Education and Self-Management for Ongoing and Newly Diagnosed (DESMOND) education programme was introduced for patients with type 2 diabetes.
2014	Biosimilar insulins increase treatment options and costs for some patients.
2015	Continuous glucose monitoring (CGM) gives real-time blood glucose readings, allowing improved management and control of diabetes.

2016	Closed-loop insulin pumps act like an artificial pancreas, with automated insulin dosages based on CGM readings.
2017	Ozempic (semaglutide) was first approved in the US for the treatment of type 2 diabetes.
2021	Ozempic was first licensed in the US as a weight-loss drug.
2025	Mounjaro (tirzepatide) was approved in the UK for obesity, type 2 diabetes and weight loss.

Glossary of Terms

Aconite is a drug derived from a poisonous plant, especially monkshood, used to relieve pain, particularly nerve pain.

Acomatrol an extract made from animal pancreases in 1908 using alcohol and saline.

Albumin a protein that balances the pressure of plasma inside and outside the cell wall.

Albuminuria refers to albumin in the urine. *Microalbuminuria* refers to a small amount of albumin in the urine—the first stage of kidney disease, while *macroalbuminuria* refers to the presence of a large amount of albumin in the urine.

Aldulab meaning 'waterwheel', this term was used by Avicenna—a physician in ancient Persian—to describe the symptoms of diabetes.

Apothecaries now known in modern times as pharmacists, made up remedies prescribed by physicians.

Arabists Persian physicians who followed Roman and Greek medical practices.

Atherosclerosis a 'furring' of the arteries, due to a build-up of fat deposits such as cholesterol.

Autoimmune attack when the body attacks itself, such as in type 1 diabetes, where insulin-producing cells are destroyed.

Autonomic neuropathy a chronic complication causing damage to autonomic nerves, which control automatic functions, such as heartbeat and the digestive system.

Aventis a pharmaceutical manufacturer who developed the insulin inhaler, in conjunction with *Pfizer* and *Nektar Therapeutics*.

Avesta a collection of ancient Persian holy writings from the sixth century A.D. These describe remedies including medical treatments and surgical techniques.

Bai Hu Jia Ren Shen Tang a herbal treatment for obesity and type 2 diabetes, used originally for symptoms seen after diagnosis.

Ba Wei Di Huang Tang Chinese medicine prescribed for weakness, fatigue and the production of copious urine.

V. Wilson, *Diabetes Ancient and Modern*, Hippocrates,
https://doi.org/10.1007/978-3-032-12454-8

Barsam an ancient Persian pear used for its glucose-lowering effects.

Biguanide a form of *guanidine*, glucose-lowering compound.

Biochemistry the chemistry of living organisms.

Bovine referring to a cow.

CGM Continuous Glucose Monitoring.

CSII Continuous Subcutaneous Insulin Infusion.

Cataplasms poultices.

Cataract describes the clouding of the lens of the eye, a chronic complication of diabetes.

Cautery use of burning Chinese wormwood oil-soaked leaves placed on the skin for the relief of pain and congestion.

Charcot disease a degenerative arthritis affecting the joints and nerves of the foot, combined with a loss of sensation, and areas of increased pressure causing hard patches of skin to form.

Chronic complications of diabetes Long-term structural changes due to high blood glucose levels that affect all areas of the body, especially causing eye disease (retinopathy), nerve damage (neuropathy), kidney disease (nephropathy), heart and circulatory problems.

Chyle term used by the seventeenth-century physician, Thomas Sydenham, to describe poor digestion and absorption in patients, which he felt was the cause of diabetes.

Collyria ancient Greek eye drops derived from verdigris (oxidised copper), used in the treatment of various eye conditions, such as cataract.

Coronary referring to the heart, and disease thereof.

Couching a treatment for cataracts where the lens of the eye is moved out of the field of vision.

Cupping an ancient technique still in use today that brings blood to the surface of the skin by suction, thought in ancient times to remove bad humours from the body.

DAFNE a structured, five-day education course for adults with type 1 diabetes, teaching how to estimate carbohydrate values and alter insulin dosage accordingly.

DCCT *Diabetes Control and Complications Trial* (1993) a groundbreaking piece of research proving that tight control on blood glucose levels reduces the risk of developing chronic complications, halting advancement of new complications, and stabilising any pre-existing complications.

Decumbiture the astrological aspects of medicine assigning signs of the zodiac to various parts of the body.

Defluxation an old term referring to excessive or abnormal outpouring of fluids, such as blood or urine, from any of the normal orifices of the body.

Depancreatised the removal of a whole or partial animal pancreas for experiment.

DESMOND a structured group education course—Diabetes Education and Self-Management for Ongoing and Newly Diagnosed—designed to help people diagnosed with type 2 diabetes to better understand and manage their condition.

Diabete an old English word that first appeared in 1425, and later became diabetes.

Diabetes (origin of) derived from the Ionian Greek word for *siphon* or *water pipe*.

Diabetes anglicus a term used by John Rollo in the eighteenth century, who did many of his experiments in England to try and determine the cause of the condition.

Diabetes insipidus a rare pituitary gland condition resulting in severe thirst and excessive urination, although the urine *does not* contain glucose.

Diabetes mellitus describes the reduced production or impaired use of the body's insulin in type 1 and type 2 diabetes, resulting in a raging thirst and frequent urination, where the urine does contain glucose.

Diabaino a term meaning *go* or *run through,* used by the Greek physician Aretaeus of Cappodocia to describe the symptoms of diabetes.

Diarrhoea urinosa a term used by the ancient Greek physician Aretaeus of Cappodocia in ancient Greece to describe the excessive urination of people with diabetes, meaning 'diarrhoea of the urine'.

Dipsakos another term formulated by Aretaeus of Cappodocia in ancient Greece referring to 'the thirsty disease'.

Dipsacus meaning 'diabetes leading to dehydration' indicated the same meaning as 'dipsakos', used by Byzantine physician, Paul of Aegina.

Dropsy an old term for congestive heart failure which describes fluid accumulation and swelling, although this term was also used to describe liver failure and malnutrition.

Dysuria term used by Aetius, a Byzantine physician, describing people with diabetes who had difficulty passing urine.

Emetics various treatments used to make a patient vomit.

Endocrine gland any gland with internal secretions, such as the pancreas, thyroid, adrenal glands, ovaries and testes.

Endocrinology the study of the endocrine system and related disorders of the endocrine glands.

Epilobium angustifolium-L a willow herb used for its laxative and purging properties, used as a treatment for diabetes.

Fei xiao translates as 'thirsting', a description of diabetes in ancient China.

Gastro relating to the stomach.

Gastroparesis a chronic condition caused by autonomic nerve damage, resulting in slow digestive transit. This in turn causes difficulty in matching the correct insulin dose to food available in the stomach and frequent low glucose levels (hypoglycaemia), followed by later high glucose levels (hyperglycaemia).

Ginkgo biloba a tree originally from Asia. The bark is used in traditional Chinese medicine to improve blood flow, especially to the extremities. This treatment is still used today for the improvement of memory.

Ginseng a Chinese herb (man-shaped root) used in a variety of treatments, such as boils, debility, fatigue, high blood glucose levels, nausea, passing large quantities of urine and sores associated with diabetes. *Panax ginseng*—a high-quality extract, improves the function of the endocrine system and control of blood glucose.

Glargine a type of long-acting insulin with no peak action times, marketed as *Lantus.*

Glucose is the major energy source for every type of cell in the body.

Glucophage the marketing name for metformin, which means 'sugar eater'.

Glycaemic control blood glucose levels within normal limits of 5–7mmol/L.

Glycogen refers to the storage of excess glucose by the liver, released into the bloodstream at times of low blood glucose.

Glycosuria refers to any excess of glucose, for example, in the urine.

Glycosylation where glucose sticks to blood proteins over the three-month lifespan of the red blood cells, the level of which can then be measured with an HbA1c test (glycosylated haemoglobin test).

Guanidine a compound that lowers blood glucose, but cannot be used as a treatment for type 2 diabetes due to its toxicity.

Gymnema sylvestre a traditional Indian tropical plant used in the treatment of diabetes.

Hepatic referring to the liver.

Hieratic a type of ancient Egyptian writing meaning 'of the priests'.

Hieroglyphic words written as pictorial figures in ancient Egyptian writing.

Histology at the level of the tissues.

Hormone an endocrine secretion that alters target body cells.

Hormone (origin) a Greek word meaning *I set in motion.*

Human Monocomponent insulin an insulin produced by Novo in 1982 derived from pigs.

Humalin is a 'human' insulin produced by *Lily* designed to mimic the action of insulin produced by the human pancreas.

Humalog a short-acting insulin lispro/lyspro.

Humours (bodily) to achieve good health, the four humours of ancient Greek medicine—blood, phlegm, yellow bile and black bile—needed to be balanced. This theory continued to be believed for more than 1500 years until the seventeenth century.

Hyperaesthesia refers to an extreme sensitivity to touch in the feet, often experienced with the chronic complication peripheral neuropathy.

Hyperglycaemia high blood glucose levels.

Hypoglycaemia low blood glucose levels where there is too much insulin working in the blood.

Immunosuppressant a steroid treatment used to stop the action of the body's immune system, such as to prevent autoimmune damage to transplanted pancreatic islet cells.

Internal suffocation prior to the discovery of insulin, this term described the effects of severe diabetic ketoacidosis, where the patient gasped for air, due to a build-up of carbonic acid from high blood glucose levels.

Insulatard a neutral insulin (also known as *Isophane*) which can be mixed in the syringe with regular insulin.

Insulin (origin) based on the Latin word for 'island'. This replaced the word 'isletin' as insulin had developed as an extract derived from the complete pancreas with no impurities.

Insuline term used in 1916 by Edward Sharpey-Schafer.

Insulin insensitivity a term used to describe the ongoing lack of effective insulin in type 2 diabetes, otherwise known as *insulin resistance.*

Insulin pump therapy (also known as CSII) the use of a continuous infusion of short-acting insulin under the skin for blood glucose management.

Insulin resistance (see *insulin insensitivity*).

Insulin sensitivity describes insulin uptake by the cells in type 1 diabetes, where there is no resistance to prevent insulin from working.

Isletin (1921) the name given to a pancreatic extract prior to the use of the word 'insulin'.

Islets (of Langerhans) named after Paul Langerhans who discovered them, these are the insulin-producing cells of the pancreas.

Isophane a neutral insulin (also known as *Insulatard*) which can be mixed with regular insulin.

Ketoacidosis the body's breakdown of fats and protein as fuel in the absence of insulin to allow the metabolism of carbohydrates. This serious health condition in diabetes requires medical attention when severe and can be detected on the patient's breath as a smell of acetone or pear drops.

Lantus a type of long-acting insulin *glargine* that has no peak working times.

Lente several long-acting insulins (*Ultralente, Lente* and *Semilente*) that can be used on their own without other insulins.

Ligation tying off to restrict flow.

Lithiasis stones (known medically as calculi) that form in the kidneys, urinary tract and gallbladder.

Lispro or Lyspro (1996) a short-acting insulin marketed as *Humalog.*

MDI multiple daily injections or multiple dose insulin.

Macrovascular the major arteries and heart.

Madhumeha an ancient Indian term describing the urine of people with diabetes as honey-like and sticky to the touch.

Mandragora a narcotic plant used in ancient Egypt as an anaesthetic during surgery.

Medicus an ancient term for doctor.

Mentha spicata used in ancient Persia, a mint extract used in the treatment of diabetes.

Metabolism (metabolise) the body's use of ingested nutrients.

Metformin a plant compound used to lower blood glucose levels in the treatment of type 2 diabetes.

Microvascular the small blood vessels within the body, such as capillaries.

Monocomponent insulin (MC) Nova produces this pure form of insulin in 1973, containing only one pancreatic component.

Morbidity the condition of having a disease or medical condition.

NICE National Institute for Health and Care Excellence.

Nektar Therapeutics a manufacturer who created an insulin inhaler in conjunction with *Pfizer* and *Aventis*.

Nephropathy describes the hardening of the kidney tissue due to continuous high blood glucose levels.

Neuropathy damage caused to the nerves by continuous high blood glucose levels.

Nordisk a Danish insulin manufacturer, formed in 1923.

NovoNordisk the combining of two Danish insulin manufacturers, formed in 1989, becoming the world's largest insulin manufacturer.

Oleum attar herbal remedy derived from oil of roses.

Pancreatine Nicolas Paulesco injected this pancreatic extract into dogs to cure their type 1 diabetes.

Pancreatitis inflammation of the pancreas, which can lead to type 1 diabetes if the islet cells become severely inflamed.

Peripheral neuropathy a complication that can manifest in two ways: *diffuse neuropathy*, affecting sensation in the hands and feet, and *distal polyneuropathy*, which can occur in a number of nerves in the hands and feet.

Pfizer the world's largest pharmaceutical manufacturer.

Pharmacea a Greek term used to describe the herbal remedies produced by physicians.

Physiology the study of organisms and how they function.

Polyuria the production and passing of large quantities of urine.

Polydipsia describes a raging thirst that cannot be quenched, due to high glucose levels.

Pompions an old word for pumpkins.

Pump Therapy see *insulin pump therapy* and *CSII.*

Principal islets the first pancreatic extract given to people with diabetes in 1907.

Prognosis describes the progression of a disease and its likely effects.

Protamine a zinc-based insulin with a delayed action time.

Pterocarpus an Indian plant used to treat high glucose levels in diabetes.

Regular insulin the name given to a fast-acting insulin solution.

Reins an ancient word for the kidneys, used in 1500 A.D.

Renaissance the new era of learning.

Renal tuberculosis a disease that is rare and usually affects young adults, resulting in weight loss, frequent urination, bladder pain and general ill health. This condition is often confused with type 1 diabetes.

Retinopathy describes several symptoms affecting vision, where the blood vessels in the eyes become larger and there are bleeds of the retina which may cause scarring and eventual blindness.

Saccharine matter describes the excessive sweetness in the organs of the digestive system in association with diabetes, mentioned by both Mathew Dobson and John Rollo.

Sanguification referring to the blood supply, as mentioned by Mathew Dobson.

Secretin a secretion of the pancreas into the small intestine, responding to stomach acid.

Shilajit decomposed plant matter in the form of a mineral pitch, derived from rocks in the Himalayas for the treatment of diabetes in ancient India.

Sodium salt.

Soluble insulin is a quick acting solution of insulin.

Sorbitol although this is the name for a sugar substitute, a different type of sorbitol is produced by the body when there is a quantity of glucose. This type of sorbitol is thought to trigger complications of diabetes in body cells.

Stem cells *Embryonic stem cells*: derived from the embryo, with the ability to create any other cell within the human body. *Adult stem cells* refer to the production of cells mainly harvested from the patient's bone marrow.

Strangury quoted by the Byzantine physician Aetius to describe passing of urine in drops rather than a constant flow.

Stroke a blockage within one or several blood vessels in the brain, which causes paralysis and speech difficulties.

Sudorific drugs used in the same way as bloodletting and emetics to make a patient vomit; inducing profuse sweating was thought to enable disease and bad humours to be expelled through the skin.

Sulfonylurea drugs first marketed in 1958 for type 2 diabetes, the drugs—*carbutamide, chlopropamide, tolbutamide* and *toldzamide*—were taken orally to reduce blood glucose levels.

Tao an ancient Chinese philosophy extolling the virtues of remaining happy and calm at all times.

Triglycerides fats within the blood.

Trigonella a traditional plant of the fenugreek family which has glucose-lowering properties.

UKPDS. The UK Prospective Diabetes Study (1998) demonstrated that blood glucose control had a direct effect on the development of eye, kidney and heart disease in people with type 2 diabetes.

Uroscopy the study of urine to diagnose diseases.

Vascularity refers to the blood vessels and the supply of blood around the body.

Veda the oldest body of literature in Hinduism, written in Sanskrit, meaning 'knowledge of life'.

Vena cava two large veins in the body known as the superior vena cava, which carries deoxygenated blood from head, neck, arms, chest to the heart, and the inferior vena cava, which transports deoxygenated blood from the legs, feet, abdomen and pelvis to the heart.

Venesection purging treatment involving cutting a vein to remove blood with the aim of balancing the humours to treat disease. (N.B.) Arteries were not used for bleeding a patient.

Viscus Persian physician Haly Abbas, used this term to mean excessive heat within the body.

Xiago ke an ancient Chinese description of diabetes, meaning 'wasting'.

Yin-yang principle the balance achieved by two mutually dependent elements, such as positive and negative.

Index

V. Wilson, *Diabetes Ancient and Modern*, Hippocrates,
https://doi.org/10.1007/978-3-032-12454-8